Healthy Waters

Positive Leadership

All Available Boats

The Best Medicine

The New Face of Aging

Positive Doctors in America

The Book of Choices

Health Politics: Power, Populism and Health

Healthy Waters

WHAT EVERY HEALTH PROFESSIONAL
SHOULD KNOW ABOUT WATER

Mike Magee, MD

Library of Congress Cataloging-in-Publication Data
Magee, Mike
Healthy Waters/Mike Magee, MD
160p. 20.32 x 12.7 cm.

ISBN 1-889793-16-7

Manufactured in Canada
First Edition

The water understands

Civilization well;

It wets my food, but prettily

It chills my life, but wittily,

It is not disconcerted,

It is not broken-hearted:

Well used, it decketh joy,

Adorneth, doubleth joy:

Ill used, it will destroy,

In perfect time and measure

With a face of golden pleasure

Elegantly destroy.

— *Ralph Waldo Emerson, 1847*

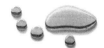

CONTENTS

We call upon the waters that rim the earth,

horizon to horizon, that flow in our rivers and streams,

that fall upon our gardens and fields,

and we ask that they teach us and show us the way.

— Chinook Indian Blessing

On September 11, 2001, along with several million other New Yorkers, I found myself on an island under attack. Several months later, I was approached to write a book that would capture a remarkable and untold story. The book, *All Available Boats,* described the largest maritime rescue since Dunkirk in World War II. It was the safe evacuation of 300,000 New York citizens in 24 hours under the expert guidance of the Coast Guard, arguably America's most under-appreciated armed force. They had sent out the call for "All Available Boats" on September 11, 2001, and coordinated the public/private flotilla's efforts in New York Harbor.

Nearly two years later, I was invited to visit the Coast Guard Academy and address its leadership on the occasion of the launch of the All Available Boats exhibit in New London, Connecticut. During the discussion I asked the leadership how it was that the Coast Guard was prepared that day to simultaneously perform three very different functions. For, on that day, their leaders had made the call for help, closed the harbor to protect against possible additional attacks and manned the piers to ensure safe loading of passengers off the island.

In response, one of their leaders said that to understand the success of that day's response, you must understand three things about the Coast Guard. First, their mission defines them as a "humanitarian force." Second, they are as prepared for peace as they are for war. And third, they honor judgment at least as much as decisiveness.

To understand these three things is to understand that when they sounded the alert on 9/11, the positive response of the boat captains in the region was ensured by a legacy of trust that extended back many years. When they closed the port, all readily complied because there existed well-established respect for the Coast Guard's authority and legitimacy. And when they manned the piers to allow safe and secure evacuation of citizens from around the world, the people complied out of respect for the Coast Guard's history of knowledge, skill and compassion in just these types of settings.

Some months later I was invited with members of the Coast Guard to recount this story to a group of water experts from the United Nations. In response to my remarks, one of the UN leaders shared the belief that the Coast Guard's influence and effectiveness was the result, in part, of its good fortune in existing at the intersection of two most powerful metaphors: Water — symbolizing life, health, hope, revitalization, purification and goodness; and vessels — representing safety, security, opportunity, fairness and transport to a better place. She asked, "What do you really know about water?"

Her question was a natural one, considering the planned announcement to come in April of 2005 of the United Nation's "Water for Life" Decade, a concentrated global focus on water as a health issue from 2005 to 2015. My embarrassed response to her question that day? "Not much!"

In exploring why this was the case, I had to admit to myself that physicians, nurses and other health care professionals (excepting the public health force) surprisingly have little connection to the policy side of water, its complexity and vast health implications. Perhaps this is because water has been positioned as an environmental issue and viewed in many quarters as ever-present and everlasting. Or perhaps it is our training, often focused on intervention and reactivity, rather than on ensuring systems and environments that promote overall wellness and the capacity to reach one's full potential. Or perhaps it is the belief that access to water, for its many varied purposes, is the responsibility of government, not the responsibility of the people or the people who care for the people.

Whatever the reason, in the wake of 9/11 and its water rescue epic, and in the wake of exposure to the Coast Guard's broad humanistic message, so in touch with our caregiving ethic, and in the face of this UN leader's very direct challenge "What do you know about water?," I decided to take action.

The first step was to work with the World Medical Association, the World Ocean Observatory and the Pfizer Medical Humanities Initiative to convene a unique gathering of water leaders and medical leaders in New York City, November 15 and 16, 2004 *(Appendix I)*. For two days, I witnessed and benefited from the introduction and cross-education between renowned water scientists on the one hand and highly respected leaders of the world's national medical, nursing and pharmacy associations on the other; and was introduced to some basic facts about water *(Appendix II)*.

The second step was to channel the energy and excitement flowing from this unique conversation into a more complete and personal exploration. This book, *Healthy Waters,* is the output of that activity. It represents an attempt to educate myself on this most important and critical health issue, and to share what I have learned with the people and the people who care for the people. It is my hope that in addressing this complex issue together, we will broaden the social context of health, engage health partners in water management and planning and advance health as the leading edge of human development.

We forget that the water cycle and the life cycle are one.

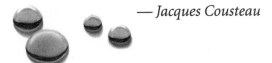

— *Jacques Cousteau*

CHAPTER 1 # Integrated Water Cycles

That water is critical to all life on our planet, humans included, is well understood by all. Much less appreciated is water's influence on the wide range of natural cycles on Earth — from food to energy to climate. In fact, water — its movement, forms, availability and transportability — has directly shaped and continues to define the future of this planet and all of its inhabitants.

We believe our planet Earth to be at least 4.3 billion years old *(Margulis and Sagan, 1986)*. That's the reading that showed up on the Sensitive High Resolution Ion Microbe Probe or SHRIMP, based on the decay rate of uranium in a Western Australian rock discovered in 1982. The oldest marine fossil was dated a half a billion years later, 3.85 billion years old, in a Greenland stone. The life form detected was not a visible fossil but rather simply a chemical residue indicating that life was once present. Victoria Bennett, its discoverer, said "we can only guess what the organism might have looked like. It was probably about as basic as life can get, but it was life nonetheless. It lived. It propagated." And it appeared just as the Earth was cooling enough to develop a solid external crust *(Bryson, 2003)*.

Scientists believe that conditions at the time were highly unsuitable for life as we know it: little oxygen, abundant hydrochloric and sulfuric acid in the atmosphere and little sunlight. Yet as Dr. Bennett stated, "…there must have been something that suited life. Otherwise we wouldn't be here" *(Bryson, 2003)*. Classic experiments in 1953 tried to mimic that ancient primordial mix. A flask of water mixed with a flask of methane, ammonia and hydrogen sulfide gasses and an electric spark thrown in delivered a thick green soup within a few days. Analysis revealed amino acids, fatty acids and sugars. Suddenly we could imagine an ancient world and our own beginning. Some fifty years later, theories have been refined. First, we believe the atmosphere was more hostile to life, a blend of nitrogen and carbon dioxide less inclined to react to energy *(Ball, 1999)*. Second, rerunning the experiment under these conditions yielded more primitive, simple amino acids. Still, as Dr. Bennett suggested, something suited life back then.

We know today that all life is built primarily around four elements, two of which are included in water. They are carbon, hydrogen, oxygen and nitrogen. Lesser amounts of sulfur, phosphorous, calcium and iron complete the palate and allow creation of three dozen plus combinations from which you can build anything that lives. And regardless of which of the many scenarios of life's beginnings you wish to embrace, water is a central feature to all *(Schopf, 1999)*.

If life began 3.8 billion years ago, little occurred over the next 2 billion years. During this time, it is felt that bacteria dominated and thrived. Very early in this period the primitive blue-green algae mastered hydrogen extraction from the water bodies, and in the process released oxygen into the atmosphere. Scientists Lynn Margulis and Dorian Sagan termed it "undoubtedly the most important single metabolic innovation in the history of life on the planet" *(Margulis and Sagan, 1986)*. Why? Because, over the first 2 billion years of Earth's life, these blue-green algae ran a photosynthesis factory that bumped up oxygen levels in our atmosphere to modern concentrations. And with that, the air and oceans, lakes and rivers changed, and a new type of complex cell, with a nucleus, organelles, multiple protective membranes, the capacity to replicate and the ability to build proteins appeared.

Life evolved and here we are. The planet Earth, its waters and its oxygen-rich atmosphere have supported our many diverse life forms — most of which thrive because their chemistry is advantaged in an oxygen- and water-rich world. We have sprung from and are dependent upon each other. The bacterium today is 75% water and, depending on type, either must have or must be shielded from oxygen to survive. We, on the other hand, have an absolute requirement for oxygen and are 65% water. What we ingest to sustain ourselves, whether steak (74% water when alive) or tomato (90% water), also require water and engage in the oxygen cycle *(Schopf, 1999)*.

Water is built through the loose bonding of water molecules. Each molecule consists of one relatively large oxygen atom connected to two smaller hydrogen atoms (H_2O). The three atoms' connection to each other is strong and resists separation. In contrast, the connection of one H_2O to another is relatively weak, with molecules pairing and unpairing billions of times a second. If one were to look at a body of water, only 15% of the H_2O molecules would be "touching" each other at any one time. This allows water to be parted easily by a boat or a swimmer or a diver. That said, the rapidity and number of recurring bonds create enough "solidity" to allow water drops to form, surface tension to exist, water bugs to walk and skipping rocks to skip on water *(Dennis, 1996)*.

Water has no taste or smell. It is formless and transparent. It can freeze and scald. Most of the water on Earth is saltwater existing in the oceans. Some 3.8 billion years ago our oceans reached their current volume, capturing and containing 97% of the planet's water in salt form. The Pacific Ocean contains 52% of this saltwater, the Atlantic Ocean 25% and the Indian Ocean 20%. This leaves a little over 3% of the saltwater for all the other oceans on Earth. The Pacific Ocean itself is massive, covering half the planet, a surface area larger than all of our land masses combined *(Figure 1.1)* *(Gordon, 2005)*.

The average ocean depth is 2.4 miles, with the deepest point some 7 miles below the surface at Mariana Trench in the Western

FIGURE 1.1

Distribution of Earth's Waters

				<1% Accessible
				• surface water
				• ground water
97% Oceans				**3% Fresh Water**

Pacific 52%	Atlantic 25%	Indian 20%	Other 3%	**2% Inaccessible**
				• snow
				• ice
Source: Gordon, 2005.				• glaciers

Pacific, 250 miles from Guam *(Broad, 1997).* As for the water itself, it only contains about 2 teaspoons of common table salt per liter, but much larger amounts of other minerals and salts that make ingestion of it by humans deadly. This is largely due to the ability of ingested salts to draw water rapidly out of our cells and trigger rapid dehydration and organ failure. That said, in certain parts of the body, we demonstrate strong affinity with the sea, creating sweat droplets and producing water tears that are remarkably similar in composition to seawater. Yet if we humans dare ingest seawater directly, we seal our own fates, for the size of the total salt load in ocean water is not small. In fact, our oceans contain a mass of salts large enough to bury all land to a depth of 500 feet. But other species seem to do quite well in seawater. In fact some estimates suggest our seas support over 30 million species spread unevenly with sites like coral reefs — rich in warmth, light and organic matter — occupying only 1% of the ocean surface but supporting 25% of the ocean's fish population *(Economist, 1998).*

The understanding that our land, its surface waters and we human inhabitants can positively or negatively impact the future of our oceans is a relatively new insight. Back in 1890, when T.H. Huxley headed a British Royal Commission examining the collapse of the herring industry, he openly ridiculed those who suggested that humans were adversely impacting the marine environment. At the time, we had a very poor understanding of the nature and volume of pollutants, of runoff and of territorial contributions to our oceans *(Kenchington, 2003)*.

Through the years, oceans have carried a mystique of being deep, dark, unexplored, impenetrable, and therefore some how safe from us. How is it possible that anything that large could be harmed? But increasingly we are viewing our ocean waters in a scientific, rather than a mythological, context. We know that seawater is 80 times as dense as air, which allows it to support tremendous biomass at low expenditures of energy. We know this medium is a comprehensive life support system. It transports, provides food and allows for reproduction. Seawater is biologically bred for life. It is a great buffer and a good solvent. It manages temperature well. A 20-degree shift in air temperature alters surface sea temperature by only a degree *(Kenchington, 2003)*.

Though ocean waters are large, they do move. They acquire particulates, good and bad, from surface land runoff and vertical upwelling from the ocean floor. In a single month, an object will travel 700 miles. The path the object will take is effected by tidal currents, weather and atmosphere and ocean geology. Life in the ocean is columnated. The upper surface is highly productive, with access to sunlight. Species feed on phytoplankton and on each other. They transport, nourish, support eggs and larvae and generally propagate. Some migrate extensively like tuna, while others are stationary like coral. Each species chooses or is chosen by a habitat. The habitat provides unique life conditions, shelter and protection. Surface conditions may vary widely, but these species are shielded compared to their terrestrial cousins. The ocean flow systems are distinctly 3-dimensional, while the land-based river and lake catchment systems are more 2-dimensional, with a relentless one-way flow to the oceans. Water may be trapped along the way due to soil or sediment buildup, flooding beyond catchment boundaries, blockages in mountain ranges or human flow diversion *(Kenchington, 2003)*.

We think we know the sea, but most of its life forms—abundant and microscopic—are invisible to us. The sea carries mystery, as fish and invertebrates move in and out of territories. Part of that mystery is the myth that the supply of life is endless, non-consumable and inexhaustible. In the latter half of the 20th century, this has been generally recognized as illogical and self-destructive. We now know that our capacity and technologically aided skills at catching fish exceed the fish communities' reproductive capacity. We know that actions in fresh water catchbasins can undermine the health of coastal ecologic systems. And we appreciate that healthy oceans are a common good. Governance on the oceans is fundamentally different from territorial oversight. Oceans are collectively owned, must be stewarded to survive and thrive and require guiding principles, laws and regulations—which in turn require enforcement.

If the amount of water stored in oceans is remarkably large, the amount contained in the atmosphere is comparably small. In fact, only .001% of Earth's water supply exists in the clouds. Most of these millions of gallons evaporate from our oceans and return to land or sea in an average 12 days. The time above does not, however, match the time below. A water molecule in the sea on average will remain as part of the sea for some 100 years. If part of a lake, the tour is somewhat less, an estimated 10 years. If landing in fertile soil, a water molecule can plan to be absorbed by a plant and re-released to the atmosphere in hours or days. But without the aid of plants, should the molecule join others as part of the ground water, there it will be for many years. If oceans deliver water, they also deliver oxygen into the atmosphere. Algae and microbes in the ocean water produce and release around 150 billion kilograms of oxygen per year *(Dennis, 1996)*.

Three quarters of the fresh water existing on Earth exists as ice, and is largely unavailable to humans. The South Pole alone contains some 6 million cubic miles of ice. Here the ice is 2 miles deep, compared with only 15 feet of ice on the North Pole. And were it all to melt, the world's oceans would rise 200 feet. By comparison, were all the atmospheric moisture to fall at once as rain, we would gain 1 inch at most. For all the ice we have, we used to have more. 25,000 years ago, 30% of our land was covered by ice. Today, 10% of the land has ice cover and 14% permafrost cover *(Shiklomanov, 1997)*.

The fresh water then, largely evaporating from ocean seawater, is constantly on the move, condensing, freezing and thawing; moving up and down, side to side, in and out. On the land it travels on the surface or below the surface at widely different speeds, forming streams and rivers with river basins and eventually draining into the seas. Along the route, some penetrates the Earth to recharge underlying aquifers or water reservoirs hidden below the Earth's crusts. Others will be drawn out at river basins to enrich soils and support agriculture, or cool turbines at manufacturing sites. At the end of the day, ground water and surface water, less than 1% of all the water on Earth, represent our potentially accessible fresh water supply. And on this fragile system, the blossom of human life survives.

It is understandable then that humankind has taken care not to wander far from our water sources. In fact civilization has carefully settled largely next to seas and river basins, supplemented these with man-made canals and has grown in numbers as a result. The water today not only sustains life but also generates food, energy and products. What happens at the river level often magnifies what is happening on the atmospheric level. For example, the regional drought that gripped Africa during the 1970s and 1980s was marked by decreased precipitation levels of 25%, but reduced annual river flows in the region by 50% *(Servat, 1998)*. Or approaching it from the other direction, in areas where sea levels rise, brackish water (a combination of sea and fresh water) moves farther and farther inland, significantly effecting the lives and livelihood of humans in these river basins.

The hydrological cycle itself, throughout human history, has been dynamic. It is now generally accepted that the assessments of the Intergovernmental Panel on Climate Change have accurately identified that global temperatures will rise 1.4°C to 5.8°C between 1990 and 2100, largely as a result of the emission of greenhouse gases — especially carbon dioxide (CO_2) *(UN, 2003)*. In response, ocean levels will rise, more energy will exist in the climate system and the global hydrological cycle will intensify. How will this be expressed? We'll see changes in amount and intensity of precipitation, in seasonal distribution and in frequency. These events in turn will lead to changes in magnitude and timing of water runoff, intensity of floods and droughts, regional water supply levels and levels of surface and ground water. In short, "terrestrial components of the hydrological cycle amplify climate input." Translation: when it comes to water, weather matters.

Precipitation across the globe is highly variable — from highs of 2,400 millimeters per year in the tropics to lows of 200 millimeters or less in the subtropics. Near the poles and at high elevations, the precipitation falls as snow, some 17,000,000,000,000 tons worldwide per year. Extremes in precipitation mean floods on the one hand and droughts on the other. Rates of evaporation are largely driven by availability of surface water exposed to air. Rates are at approximately 2,000 millimeters per year in the subtropics, decreasing to about 500 millimeters per year as you approach the poles *(Shiklomanov, 2002)*.

Soil is a significant reservoir for water. Amounts are not only driven by the rates of precipitation and evaporation but also by soil type and depth, vegetation, topography and seasonality. Within a small area, levels of water absorption and soil moisture are highly variable. The top two meters contain the majority of the moisture, estimated at 16,500 cubic kilometers *(Korzun, 1974)*. Significant water also collects in subterranean spaces. The presence of stored ground water is often revealed by surface springs. The supply of fresh water throughout human existence has greatly exceeded our ability to access it. That said, ground water has been critical to human development. In the past 50 years, with advances in drilling and pump technology, ground water has rapidly become the world's "most extracted raw material." Whether city (70% of the piped water supply of the European Union) or rural (sub-Saharan Africa), manufacturing or agriculture (Asia's green agriculture revolution), ground water is a major driver in human development as we enter the 21st century.

The challenge remains how best to scientifically manage this raw material to ensure long-term sustained development. This requires a better understanding of how the ground water systems function, their recharge processes and their relationships to surface water bodies. It also means managing and protecting the purity and integrity of the resource, a knowledge of the geology, better monitoring of ground water levels and real-time data of depth, flows and extraction levels. But for the effort, the rewards are high. Ground water is the predominant strategic reservoir on Earth, some 30% of the global fresh water total and 98% of the drinkable and potentially accessible supply. And compared with surface water, there is very little loss to direct evaporation *(Shiklomanov, 1998)*.

While humankind can greatly benefit from wise management of ground water sources, it can equally place itself at great risk by mismanagement of this resource. From 1950 to 1970, the developed world invested heavily in ground water exploration. Over the following two decades, the developing world weighed in as well. Today, ground water provides 50% of the world's drinkable water, 40% of that used by industry and 20% of that used for agricultural irrigation *(Zektser and Margat, 2004)*. Its economic benefits include local availability, drought resistance and good quality. Approximately 1.2 billion urban citizens worldwide subsist on well, borehole or spring water. In countries like India, every sector is reliant *(FAO. Aquastat, 2002)*. 80% of India's rural domestic supply and 70% of its agriculture output is the result of ground water extraction. In some areas, such as the North China Plain and among some 100 Mexican aquifers, extraction rates of 5 to 10 cubic kilometer per year (km^3/year) are clearly not sustainable. In such areas, urban needs already compete with those of agriculture, and lack of wastewater management and careful integrated planning further complicates the modern picture *(UN, 2003)*.

As water seeps into ground water aquifers, it also seeps out through watercourses, wetlands and coastal zones. Recharge rates are highly variable and affected by changes in surface vegetation, surface water diversion, changing water table levels and climate cycles. Sustainability issues include inefficient use, social inequity, unsustainable extraction, icy weather reductions, aquifer damage, land compaction and ecosystem damage. All of these are under human control. Aquifers are far more resistant to contamination than are surface water bodies. But once contaminated, aquifer damage is difficult to reverse.

As with most enlightened policy, good planning and prevention pays off. Sound system design, proper land use rights, ongoing investment in technology, stakeholder participation and careful monitoring, design and operation are critical. But what's unique about water is that water flows. And in flowing, it crosses multiple jurisdictional borders. So proper management and planning require intergovernmental cooperation. This holds true to some extent for surface water supplies as well. River basin networks cover 45% of the Earth's land and nourish locations that support 60% of our global population. There are over 15 million lakes and reservoirs on the planet, though the 145 largest hold 168,000 cubic kilometer (km^3) of water or 95% of the total lake water on Earth. Of this, approximately half is fresh and half is saltwater. The Caspian Sea, one of the world's largest lakes, contains 91% of the Earth's inland saltwater *(Figure 1.2) (Shiklomanov, 2005)*.

FIGURE 1.2

Global Surface Water Supply Highlights

	· River basin networks: – Cover 45% of land. – Support 60% of population.
	· 15 million+ lakes: – Half are fresh water, half are saltwater. – The 145 largest hold 95% of the Earth's total lake water.
Source: Shiklomanov, 2005.	**· Manmade structures:** – There are 47,655 large dams on the planet, and more than 800,000 smaller ones. – There are 633 large reservoirs on the Earth.

Where there are lakes, there are dams. These are built for flood control, to support irrigation, to replace over-consumption of ground water and to support recreation, among other things. As of 2000, there were 47,655 large dams (a height of more than 15 meters) and more than 800,000 smaller ones. Dams have been around for at least 5,000 years. In 2004, some 300 dams over 60 meters in height were under construction. More are expected in the future to meet demand. In addition, there are 633 large reservoirs with a total volume of 5,000 km^3 (63% of the total reservoirs' storage volume), which capture approximately 40% of the Earth's fresh runoff water and 30% of river sediment. The reservoirs not only capture surface water but also increase surface area evaporation by some 200 km^3 of water per year *(Figure 1.3) (Hoeg, 2000)*.

By comparison, river volume of surface water is quite small, but highly strategic. In many parts of the world, river water is the most accessible and certainly most over utilized and stressed fresh water resource. While most rivers reach the ocean, some do not, including those draining into the Caspian Sea (a lake), the Arabian peninsula, central Australia, North Africa and Middle and Central Asia. These feed 20% of the Earth's land surface but contain

FIGURE 1.3

Dams

Use:	
	• Dams are used for power, water reservoirs, industry use, irrigation, and flood mitigation.
Number:	
	• There are over 47,000 large dams worldwide.
	• 50% of all large rivers have a dam.
Producers:	
	• The largest dam builders today are India and China.
Durability:	
	• Most dams are functional 40 years later.

Source: Hoeg, 2000.

only 2% of its fresh water runoff *(UNESCO, 1993)*. In contrast, the Amazon River in Latin America, the world's longest river, captures 16% of the world's runoff; and the Amazon, Ganges (India), Congo (Central Africa), Yangtze (China) and Orinoco (Venezuela) together capture and transport 27% of the runoff, all to the sea. The average total flow per year from land to sea for all rivers is 42,800 km^3. This runoff occurs mainly (60%–70%) in spring and early summer. Most flooding occurs during this time and carries large amounts of sediment and organic material with it. While large year-to-year variations in flow occur, careful studies over 65 years show no significant trends.

Before extensive human interventions, surface water quality varied as a result of land use, geology climate, biologic activities and geography. But today there are few examples of natural surface water bodies. The impact of industry, agriculture, wastewater mismanagement and urbanization has affected the chemical composition of average river water. Comparing natural to actual water concentrations of various chemicals reveals the human impact on the chemical nature of our surface water *(Figure 1.4) (Meybeck, 1979)*.

The human touch has left its mark. From industrial heavy metals to acid rain, from leaking storage tanks, accidental spillage and domestic sewage to municipal waste and agro-industrial effluent,

FIGURE 1.4

Human Impact on Chemical Composition
of Surface Water
Concentration (milligrams/liter)

	NATURAL	ACTUAL
Calcium	13.4	14.7
Magnesium	3.4	3.7
Sodium	5.2	7.2
Potassium	1.3	1.4
Chlorine	5.8	8.3
Sulfate	8.3	11.3
Bicarbonate	52.0	53.0
Silicon Dioxide	10.4	10.4
Dissolved Solids	99.6	110.1

Source: Meybeck, 1979.

people and water definitely do mix. Besides affecting the quality of drinking water, secondary impacts have become common. For example, the discharge of organic material, high in nitrogen and phosphorous, into surface water fosters abnormal and explosive plant growth, depleting oxygen and affecting the entire ecosystem and the life forms it supports. Twentieth century ecosystem degradation has resulted in the loss of 50% of our wetlands and 20% of our fresh water species *(Figure 1.5) (UN, 2003).*

FIGURE 1.5

20th Century Ecosystem Degradation

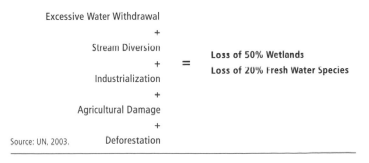

Excessive Water Withdrawal
+
Stream Diversion
+
Industrialization
+
Agricultural Damage
+
Deforestation

=

**Loss of 50% Wetlands
Loss of 20% Fresh Water Species**

Source: UN, 2003.

The river waters cannot be separated from solid and particulate sediment. Some of this exists in the riverbeds, disturbed and activated by flows and floods. Much exists as suspended matter, actively in motion. In fact, more than 50 billion tons of suspended sediment is carried by river waters to the oceans each year *(Walling and Webb, 1996)*. What lands in surface water and ground water bodies is increasingly a function of human action and planning. For example, creation of solid surfaces increases volume and rate of runoff, downstream flooding and human chemical deposits into surface water. Over-mining of ground water impacts water levels and the capacity to live off the land in stressed locations around the world. High surface runoff carries with it expanded sewage runoff in urban environments. Poor liquid waste disposal and hazardous chemical spills travel rapidly above the ground and easily penetrate below the ground in many locations. And as these collective actions impact lakes, rivers and streams, habitats and species diversity decline.

There is then a natural, interconnected and crucial water cycle upon which all life on Earth depends. Humans have always required a dependable water supply to survive and thrive. As we have grown in numbers and in concentration, as we have built and infiltrated among and, at times, in opposition to other life forms, we have created future health challenges that must now be addressed. To do so, each of us must better understand the nature of water and its relations to weather, ecosystems, agriculture, industry, urban planning, sanitary systems and value of Integrated Water Resource Management (IWRM).

For many of us, water simply flows from a faucet,

and we think little about it beyond this point of contact.

We have lost a sense of respect for the wild river,

for the complex workings of a wetland,

for the intricate web of life that water supports.

We have been quick to assume rights to use water

but slow to recognize obligations to preserve

and protect it... in short, we need a water ethic —

a guide to right conduct in the face of

complex decisions about natural systems

we do not and cannot fully understand.

— Sandra Postel,

Last Oasis: Facing Water Scarcity

CHAPTER 2 The Water Crisis

In the beginning of the 21st century, we find ourselves awakening to a water crisis. The signs are everywhere. 25,000 humans a day die from lack of food and water. 6,000 lives are lost each day to waterborne diseases *(UN, 2003)*. Such losses reflect more than disordered supply and demand, and more than inequitable distribution or lack of access to this most essential resource. Rather, they reflect a lack of will and a lack of knowledge to manage water use and abuse in an intelligent way.

That a water crisis is on the radar screen is undeniable. The United Nations Millennium Declaration in 2000 directed members to "stop the unsustainable exploitation of water resources by developing water management strategies at the regional, national and local levels, which promote both equitable access and adequate supplies." But saying it is not doing it, and to advocate and collaborate, we need some very basic understanding of the complex relationship between ourselves, our water and our planet.

For humans, water is not a luxury, but a necessity — for drinking, for food, for washing, for producing products, for generating energy, for moving people, for moving goods, for progress. Yet as critical as it is, most of the peoples of the developed and developing world alike know little about water as a resource and in general take water for granted.

It is probable that most of the world's citizens never heard the UN alarm in 2000 *(UNEP, 2000)* that "the world water cycle seems unlikely to be able to adapt to the demands that will be made of it in the coming decades" *(Figure 2.1)*. Fewer still have read the Earth Summit in

FIGURE 2.1

Humans and Water Usage

	• Between 1900 and 2000, the human population increased 300%, while water consumption grew 600%.
Source: UNEP, 2000.	• Between 2000 and 2020, a 40% increase in human water consumption is predicted. During the same period, a 17% increase in agricultural water consumption is expected.

Rio de Janeiro's words from 1992: "Water is needed in all aspects of life. The general objective is to make certain that adequate supplies of water of good quality are maintained for the entire population of this planet, while preserving the hydrological, biological and chemical functions of ecosystems, adapting human activities within the capacity limits of nature and combating vectors of water-related diseases."

Proclamations and warnings tend to poorly communicate the complexity of the water crisis issue. On one level it is an equity and justice issue. Water is not evenly accessible. For example, the Middle East has 5% of the world's population but only 1% of its water *(Health Politics, 2004)*. Water consumption of a child in the developed world is up to 50 times greater than a child in the developing world. Women are unequally disadvantaged by water scarcity as they do the majority of water transport in developing countries, require it for household and agricultural responsibilities, and suffer unequally from maternal-fetal diseases when it is scarce or soiled.

Health and hygiene issues are inseparably tied to water. The United Nations stated in 2000, "clean water alone leads only to minor health improvements in the absence of personal hygiene and adequate sanitation." 6,000 deaths, mostly of children, each day are due to water-related diseases *(Figure 2.2)*. Water touches, in one way or another, every diarrheal and infectious disease. When it is scarce, famine, malnutrition and dehydration ensure compromised hosts, creating an explosive environment for HIV, malaria and tuberculosis. Poor policy impacts safety, privacy, convenience and dignity. Bad

FIGURE 2.2

Causes of Death in Children Under Age 5

	Neonatal Disorder	**37%**
	Acute Respiratory Infection	**19%**
	Diarrhea	**17%**
	Malaria	**8%**
	Measles	**4%**
	HIV/AIDs	**3%**
Source: WHO/UNICEF, 2005.	Other	**12%**

FIGURE 2.3

Water Disease Triangle

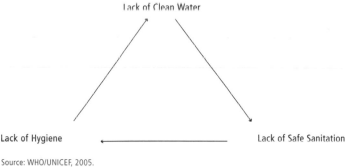

Lack of Clean Water

Lack of Hygiene   Lack of Safe Sanitation

Source: WHO/UNICEF, 2005.

decisions regarding sanitation lead to bad water. Bad water leads to poor health, low productivity and the loss of hope *(Figure 2.3) (WHO/UNICEF, 2005)*.

An examination of poverty reveals poor water access as a major determinant. Access to water is critical to basic needs, nutrition, general health and securing a livelihood. Of the seven key challenges facing the global community according to the 2003 UN Development Report, safe water is well-represented. In addition, the other obstacles — life expectancy, health services, underweight children under age five and literacy — all rely on adequate clean water supplies to be addressed.

The Organization for Economic Cooperation and Development (OECD) in its Poverty Guidelines in 2001 states, "poverty, gender and environment are mutually reinforcing, complementary and cross-cutting facets of sustainable development." And from the UN, "One of the main characteristics of poverty is now seen as vulnerability...This includes both shocks (sudden changes such as natural disasters, war or collapsing market prices) and trends (for example, gradual environmental degradation, oppressive political systems or deteriorating terms of trade). Many such vulnerabilities are related to water resources (for example, health threats, droughts or floods, cyclones and pollution). The need to integrate vulnerability reduction into water policies (and in particular the links between water policies, disaster mitigation and climate changes) is being increasingly considered" *(UN, 2003)*.

The message, then, is that water must be addressed in an integrated way. So, for example, the UN's Vision 2015 standards place side by side decreasing by one half the proportion of people without access to hygienic sanitation facilities, and reducing by one half the proportion of people without sustainable access to adequate quantities of affordable and safe water. They also target 2025 as the date when nations should "provide water, sanitation and hygiene for all." An integrated view is also reflected in balancing the need for food, raw materials and products for sustained development in concert with water preservation. Clearly, poor planning can pull everyone and everything down. Whether it be wastage precipitated by deforestation, erosion and flooding, or damage to surface or ground water by pollution, little margin for error exists to accommodate human ignorance. To advance together as a human population we must address poverty, hunger, education, gender inequality, child mortality, maternal mortality and infectious diseases.

When handled wisely, water sources are renewable. They are also variable, by geography and by seasons. For example, total renewable water per capita per year varies from a high of 10,767,857 m^3/cap/yr in Greenland to a low of 276 m^3/cap/yr in Israel *(FAO, Aquastat, 2002)*. Planning must account for this variability. Resources for most of the world's water needs — for drinking, agriculture, industry, waste removal and preservation of ecosystems — literally "drops out of the sky" in the form of precipitation. The water moves vertically and horizontally in a water cycle. This water manages, mainly by diverting as runoff or accessing ground sources, to support our consumption. It is estimated that 26% of precipitation and 54% of accessible runoff is now accessed by humans. And usage rates, fueled by population growth, life style changes and expansion of agriculture, industry and urbanization, are projected to increase substantially. By 2050, one in four worldwide will experience chronic or recurring shortage of fresh water. 2 billion are already impacted one way or another by water shortage in 40 countries. 1.1 billion don't have enough clean water to drink and 2.4 billion have no sanitary facilities, making clean water even less likely. In addition, progress will require cooperation, as rivers cross national boundaries. Worldwide, 263 river basins cross at least one border, and these rivers service over 40% of the world's population *(UN, 2003)*.

What water we have is frequently polluted. Human waste, some two million tons a day, discarded directly into surface water basins, is the most common culprit. Agricultural pesticides and fertilizers as well as industrial chemicals contribute as well. Together, man-made deposits of one sort or another ensure that 50% of the citizens in developing nations receive water that is unacceptable for ingestion. In it, you will find fecal bacteria, organic chemicals, heavy metals, nitrates and phosphates from farms and sediment resulting from poor land management *(WHO/UNICEF, 2000)*.

The conversion has been rapid and recent. In Asia, over three decades, suspended solids have increased by a factor of four and human waste by a factor of three. With pollution comes disease, accessed through unhealthy behaviors. For example, in Varanasi, India, a sacred site on the Ganges River, 60,000 people bathe in the polluted waters each day *(CSE, 1999)*. Asia as well is at the epicenter of water-related disasters, accounting for 40% of all such events. Worldwide, there were approximately 2,500 water-related disasters with 665,000 deaths between 1991 and 2000 *(UN, 2003)*. The year 2000 had 153 flood events, and the tsunami in 2004 alone resulted in 220,000 deaths *(Health Politics, 2005)*.

On the supply side then, we have inherited a renewable resource, if wisely managed in an integrated fashion. But the supply of water is only as good as its quality and reliability. As global populations rise, all other things being equal, supplies of water per capita fall. In fact, available water per person declined by one-third between 1970 and 1990. Currently, population growth is slowing down with the total number of people worldwide expected to increase from 6.1 billion in 2001 to about 9.3 billion by 2050 and there remain stable. So even though our rate of growth is declining, we still must assimilate a population that will be 52% larger by 2050 than it is now. Translating these numbers to projected water realities leads experts to predict that 7 billion people in 60 countries will be dealing with water scarcity by 2050. This is 75% of our future global population. Were we to embrace the most optimistic projections, 2 billion in 48 nations, or 22%, will be water-scarce *(UNFPA, 2002)*.

As these growing numbers must drink, so must they eat. And while our daily water requirement to survive is less than 3 liters, it takes about 3,000 liters of water to grow our daily food requirement *(UN, 2005b)*. This means more demand for agricultural yield, drier season planting and more exploitation of both surface and ground waters. The population will also require increased energy. Hydropower is a significant resource for developed and developing nations, generating 70% and 30% respectively of the total hydroelectric output worldwide over the past few decades. Most water consumption related to hydroelectric plants comes from evaporation from the surface of the large reservoirs. In the future, use of hydroelectric power will grow, especially in the developing world, which has only tapped 15% of its total potential. Though substantial amounts of water are used for cooling and the chemical process, most is returned to the watershed without consequences, unless significant water temperature variations are not properly managed. Overall, the generation of hydroelectric energy is considered by most to be environmentally benign *(UN, 2003)*.

As hydroelectric production grows, so will urbanization. By 2025, 58% of the world's population will be urban. The greatest increases will occur in Asia. For example, south-central Asia is projected to grow in urban population from some 400 million to 1 billion by 2030. By that time, about 3 billion citizens will be rural and 4 billion will be urban. This influx of people to the cities will further stress water supply and sanitation infrastructure. This will lead to predictable over-exploitation of aquifers and falling water levels. Pollution, unchecked, will further compromise the usefulness of what water there is, sending many to private vendors, taxing a vulnerable population with high water prices *(UNFPA, 2002)*.

As we urbanize, we will continue to industrialize. Polluting industries are also fast growth industries. For example, paper and steel industries in Latin America are growing at twice the rate of the local economy. Wastewater from factories contains high levels of suspended solids that line and suffocate waterway life. Organic material competes for oxygen, and heavy metals interfere with reproduction of species. Occasional industrial accidents can be devastating to water supply. A single fire in a Swiss pesticide plant in 1986 shut down water supply for 1,000 kilometers downstream for days. New technology may offer some protection, providing remote sensing and active and effective monitoring. We can expect in the near future better drilling and extraction of ground water, better transport and improved decentralization. Technology will also improve efficiency of drinking, bathing and sanitation systems *(UN, 2003)*.

It will have to, in order to countercheck demand, driven in part by the belief that water is a right, to be used without limit or common sense; by expanded needs for agriculture and manufacturing; and by globalization, urbanization and tourism. In 1970, less than 8% of citizens from developed nations had visited a developing nation. The number now sits at 29% and is rising. This of course carries economic benefits, but also consumes a disproportionate share of water and public infrastructure resources for tourism. In the Caribbean islands, 80% to 90% of hotel sewage in 1994 was deposited directly, untreated, into coastal waters. And a single 18-hole golf course consumes more than 2.3 million liters of water a day *(UN, 2003)*.

Finally, we must increasingly consider climate change. It is now universally recognized that increased carbon dioxide and other greenhouse gases are driving significant global climate changes. These are projected to yield significant increases in precipitation from 30° North and 30° South due to expanded evaporation. Tropical and subtropical regions in contrast will see rainfall become less common and more erratic. Most agree now that there will be climate change, but where, when and how much are up for dispute. That said, many believe that arid areas — currently most water-stressed — are likely to experience declines, not rises, in water levels due to climate variation. There is also general concern that these changes will result in an increase in the number and severity of water-related disasters, including floods, droughts, mudslides, typhoons and cyclones *(Abramovitz, 2001)*. A study in 2000 projected that 20% of our future water scarcity would be the result of climate variations, and 80% would result from population growth and its secondary effects *(Vorosmarty, 2000)*.

What is indisputable is that absent careful, planned and consistent action, our water crisis will worsen. The Conference on Water in Dublin in 1992 layed out these principles:

1. Fresh water is a finite and vulnerable resource, essential to sustain life, development and the environment.
2. Water development and management should be based on a participatory approach, involving users, planners and policy makers at all levels.
3. Women play a central part in the provision, management and safeguarding of water.
4. Water has an economic value in all its competing uses and should be recognized as an economic good.

The 1994 UN Commission on Sustainable Development said it this way:

"While in the past there was a tendency to regard water problems as being regional in nature, there is growing recognition that their increasingly widespread occurrence is quickly adding up to a crisis of global importance."

And in 1998:

"It is important that consideration of equitable and responsible use of water becomes an integral part in the formulation of strategic approaches to integrated water management at all levels, in particular in addressing the problems of people living in poverty."

And two years later, in 2000, seven challenges were defined with four more added later:

1. Meet basic needs: Provide access to safe and sufficient water and sanitation for basic human needs; and empower women in this process.
2. Secure the food supply: Efficiently use water for food production, and equally allocate water for food production.
3. Protect ecosystems: Ensure the integrity of ecosystems.
4. Manage risk: Provide security from flood, drought, pollution and water hazards.
5. Share water resources: Encourage peaceful cooperation and synergies whenever possible.

6. Value water: Manage water in a manner that reflects its economic, social, environmental and cultural values in all uses with a move towards pricing to reflect true cost, but ensuring basic provision for the poor and vulnerable.
7. Govern water wisely: Ensure good governance involving the public and stakeholders in integrated water management.
8. Water and cities: Manage distinct challenges to water and sanitation that come with urbanization.
9. Water and industry: Manage needs and water quality, considering economic needs, energy needs and competing interests.
10. Water and energy: Recognize that water is vital for all forms of energy production.
11. Ensure the knowledge base: Provide decision makers with the knowledge necessary to ensure good water policy and management.

And finally in 2002, the call for sustained development in Africa with specific policies, strategies and real commitments in six specific areas:

1. Access to clean water and sanitation.
2. Focus on secure food supply and income generation.
3. Advance Integrated Water Resource Management (IWRM) locally and globally.
4. Ensure water-related disaster prevention, mitigation and management.
5. Empower capacity building with a special focus on equity and gender sensitivity.
6. Encourage pro-poor water governance and water policies.

There is, then, an undeniable momentum gathering within the international community. Since water touches literally everyone and everything, it is the logical beginning point and transcendent metaphor for sustainable development. Water is more broadly viewed today as a potentially renewable, but threatened resource. Water's complex interfaces are increasingly evident, and its value increasingly understood. Supplying safe, clean water has a price, as does wasting or fouling this critical resource. Its supply must rise to meet its forecast population demand. Water scarcity is a crisis today, with solutions that cannot wait until tomorrow.

Water sustains all.

— Thales of Miletus, 600 B.C.

CHAPTER 3 Water and Health

Over the past decade, the definition of health has taken on broader dimensions. Health is not as limited as the health systems themselves, nor is it synonymous with the wide range of caregivers nor the tactics they utilize to detect and fight disease. Rather, today, health for the individual is a state of well-being that would allow each man or woman, each girl or boy, to reach her or his full potential as a human being. In its 1948 Constitution, the World Health Organization (WHO) defined health as "a complete state of physical, mental and social well-being, and not merely the absence of disease or infirmity" *(WHO, 2002)*. Health on the larger national scale has become the leading edge of development, and as such eventually touches all other sectors, including food, energy, industry, ecosystems, cities and — of course — water.

As we have broadened our vision of health, the full meaning of water to the human race has begun to reveal itself. In the most concrete terms, our dependency on water is indisputable. We are literally 65% water. The average human consumes 2.3 liters of water a day — a half a liter goes to sweat, .3 liters is released through breathing, and 1.5 liters are eliminated as waste. If we lose 1% of our water, we become thirsty. If we lose 5%, a mild fever develops. Lose 10%, and we are immobilized. And if we lose 12%, we die *(Figure 3.1) (Swanson, 2001)*. Our cells are able to communicate with each other through a network of nerve signals and hormone packages that travel on our bodies' complex internal rivers and streams. Our various organs fulfill their responsibilities with the help of nutrients arriving within blood, lymph and other liquid

FIGURE 3.1

Humans Need Water

We are composed of 65% water.
• The average individual consumes 2.3 liters of water a day.
• This water is released as:
− .5 liters of sweat,
− .3 liters of respiration and
− 1.5 liters of urine/feces.
The effects of dehydration vary according to how much water is lost:
• 1% dehydration causes thirst.
• 5% dehydration causes fever.
• 10% dehydration causes loss of mobility.
• 12% dehydration causes death.

Source: Swanson, 2001.

secretions. Our bodies release toxins and poisons by transporting them through liver, kidneys and colon. Our fluids are in constant motion, elements added and removed, to energize functions, maintain order, support conscious and unconscious actions and sustain life.

Beyond staying alive, individuals and families require water to maintain a stable healthy household. With 5 liters a day, an individual can barely survive. With 20 liters a day, a family can marginally complete tasks that ensure health and sanitation. With 50 liters a day, one can lower the public health risks associated with poor hygiene; can clean clothes on-site near home; and can have fresh water available in proximity to living quarters. With 100 to 200 liters per day, you are most likely living in a developed economy, with multiple taps inside the home, shielded largely from hygiene-related illness *(Figure 3.2) (UN, 2003)*.

The World Health Organization says that 75 liters of water a day is necessary to protect against household disease, and 50 liters a day necessary for basic family sanitation. But individual consumption varies widely around the globe. A member of the Masai Tribe in Africa survives on approximately 4 liters per day, while a typical resident of Los Angeles, California uses 500 liters per day *(Swanson, 2001)*.

FIGURE 3.2

WHO Standards:
Access to Water

		DISTANCE	VOLUME/ CAPITA/ DAY	HEALTH RISK
	Optimal	**in-house, multiple taps**	**100–200 liters**	**very low**
	Good	**on property, 1 tap**	**50 liters**	**low**
	Basic	**less than 1 km away**	**20 liters**	**high**
Source: UN, 2003.	Poor	**more than 1 km away**	**5 liters**	**very high**

For many years, the clearest connection between water failure and poor health has been water-borne diseases *(WHO, 2002)*. In 2005, 6,000 people, mostly young children, will die each day from diarrheal and infectious diseases. Adequate amounts of clean drinking water and basic sanitation services would dramatically impact these numbers. Improved systems would reduce disease burden by 17%. Perfect piped water and sanitation systems would decrease it by 70%. But the reality is that 1.1 billion people lack access to improved water and 2.4 billion —42% of the world's population — lack access to improved sanitation *(UN, 2005a)*.

One half of all hospital beds in the developing world are occupied by individuals suffering from water-borne diseases. If you are part of a village of 1,000 in Africa, here's what you'll see. Over 600 will have no access to a latrine; 20 on any given day will suffer from diarrhea, with 15 under the age of 5. For a family of six, hauling water from a distant location will eat up 3 hours a day. Most children will not have time between water hauling and chores to attend school. Conditions will be filthy and disease will spread rapidly. As desperate as a situation like this can be, it is by no means hopeless. A 2005 study demonstrated that improved water supply reduced death from diarrheal illness up to 25%. Better hygiene, including education and promotion of disposal of infant feces, hand washing and safe storage and protection of domestic water supply, reduced diarrheal cases 45%. And household water treatment, for example chlorination and proper home water storage, decreased cases by up to 39% *(UN, 2003)*.

That said, the real difference in the past five years is the context within which we consider the water challenge. It is not generally accepted, nor properly understood, that success with water will speed achievement of seven additional United Nations Millennium Development Goals. These include helping to "eradicate extreme poverty and hunger; achieving universal primary education; promoting gender equality and empowering women; reducing child mortality and improving maternal health; combating HIV/AIDS, tuberculosis, malaria and other diseases; ensuring environmental sustainability and developing a global partnership for development."

"Squalor, poverty, and disease": These are the enemies and the reflections of poor water policy. And the targets above appear financially feasible with an excellent return on investment. A well-documented WHO study says it would cost an additional $11.3 billion a year. In return there are $7 billion in direct health care savings, $3.5 billion in productivity increases, $3.5 billion in family earnings preserved by averting untimely death and $63 billion in time savings attributable to immediately accessible water and sanitation. In sum, the $11.3 billion investment delivers a $77 billion payback *(Figure 3.3) (UN, 2003)*.

FIGURE 3.3

**Water Development:
A Sound Investment**

Meeting the UN Millennium Goals for improved water and sanitation would result in:
- An annual investment of $11.3 billion.
- An annual savings of $77 billion, including:
  – An additional 272 million school attendance days.
  – An additional 320 million productive work days.
  – An additional 1.5 billion healthy days for children under age 5.

Source: UN, 2003.

HEALTHY WATERS

Definitions of what is "safe water" and "basic sanitation" have been all over the map. The WHO and UNICEF clearly have defined what is and is not acceptable *(WHO/UNICEF, 2005)*. For water, unprotected wells and springs and uncertified vendor water, tanker truck water and surface water are unimproved approaches. In contrast, piped water, public taps, boreholes (synonym for drilled wells, especially outside North America), protected wells and springs, rainwater collection and certified bottled water are improved techniques. For sanitation, public or shared latrines, hanging latrines, bucket latrines and absent facilities are unacceptable. Flush systems to sewers, septic tank or latrine, ventilated improved pit latrines, and pit latrines with stalls and composting toilets all represent advances.

Beyond these standards, it's critical to understand that creating infrastructure for water and sanitation implies continued investment to maintain these systems. Otherwise, the gains are short-lived. For example, estimates in Africa are that 30% of the water and sanitation systems do not function properly. In Asia, the estimate is 20%. Within individual countries, extreme outliers have more than 50% of facilities requiring repair or replacement. One additional point: one can no longer presume that surface and ground water are safe. This requires that sufficient investment and systems be in place to regularly sample, analyze and monitor water quality *(WHO/UNICEF, 2000)*.

Water management or mismanagement impacts multiple generations. For the very young, the burden of disease is extraordinarily high, with 90% of water-related deaths occurring in children age 0 to 4. For those age 5 to 14 years, disease, domestic responsibility for hauling water or working the fields or lack of private latrines, especially for schoolgirls, translates into poor school attendance and a limited future *(WHO, 2002)*.

In 2002, 500 million of these school-aged children lacked proper sanitation and 230 million had compromised water. Worldwide, 24% of boys and 28% of girls did not attend primary school in

2002. Regional numbers were worse. 39% of boys and 44% of girls in the least-developed countries did not attend primary school *(WHO/UNICEF, 2005)*. This then is a double hit. Lacking education, lifespan options contract. But in addition, one valuable source of health education, including basic hygiene — the school — is no longer a community platform for programs. In some locations, the strategic connection between health and school is being fully leveraged. The School Sanitation and Hygiene Education Program (http://www.unicef.org/wes/index_schools.html) is a good example. In Nigeria, teachers are prepared in life skills education, parent involvement, village participation in hygiene and sanitation projects and formation of children hygiene clubs. The result: a 20% increase in school enrollment and 77% decrease in water-borne worms *(UN, 2003)*.

For adults, women continue to literally "carry the load" for inaccessible water, and both men and women are made more susceptible to diseases like HIV/AIDS, malaria and tuberculosis by lack of water and under-nourishment. And as they pass age 60, this susceptibility grows with each year. The clear reality and immediate impact of poor water and sanitation is lost productivity and work. Life comes to a halt as families drudge buckets of water for miles to support planting, cleaning and preparing food. If they are fortunate enough to survive beyond the age of 60, they will join the ranks of 1 billion global citizens by 2025. By then, water-borne infection death rates in those over age 60 in the developing world will exceed water-borne infection death rates of the age 0 to 5 population in their countries. This reflects elder susceptibility to water-borne pathogens arising from declining hygiene, poorly maintained services, absent vigilance, more underlying chronic disease, reduced immune function, under-nutrition and increased poverty with increasing age *(WHO/UNICEF, 2005)*.

For women around the world, water is a lifelong health headache. To begin with, they and their daughters are the source and utilizers of most water. It has fallen on women to provide most water and food, to support bathing, cooking, household hygiene and cleansing of infants, children, the sick and the elderly. In India, the national cost to women of fetching water is estimated at 150 million women workdays per year. On average they walk 6 kilometers a day carrying 20 liters of water. Sick children consume an enormous portion of maternal productivity. Pregnancy presents special demands, and poor water and sanitation places mother and fetus at risk before, during and after birth. As a target for HIV/ AIDS, women are often innocent victims. Demands never stop for women. Household gardens must be seeded, watered and tended; livestock fed, milked and harvested. Even care and repair of dwellings with homemade bricks and mud are water-dependent. While women are charged with gathering and wisely managing water in most of the world, their voices and opinions, until recently, have been excluded from overall water and sanitation management policy making. As a result, in many communities the best knowledge source has been sequestered, and the knowledge itself lost to the community (UN, 2003).

If we were to fully access women and ask what would be of greatest help, what would they say? First, meet basic requirements for sanitation. Second, significantly increase access to safe water. Third, focus on promoting basic hygiene education. Fourth, adopt simple techniques for disinfecting drinking and cooking water in the home, including chlorination, disinfection and filters. Fifth, adequately resource health care. Of course, to respond would require governments to establish the right policies, planning and follow-through, which in turn requires enlightened legislation, regulation, strong institutions, well-trained workers, right choices in technology, excellent educational and behavioral programming and continuous learning and improvement.

Integrated responses are very specific and customized from a cultural point of view. However various lessons and principles are highly transferable. For example, Nepal has customized a UNICEF program on sanitation, incorporating it into their school health curriculum. It has five major components, including hygiene habit-formation, building sanitary facilities at schools, maintaining these facilities in working order, organizing extracurricular events around good sanitation and transferring learning from school to community. In Peru, the emphasis has been squarely focused on hand washing, with significant reductions in illness. Their approach: form a local team, enlist community leaders, pretest promotional/ educational materials, develop appropriate measures and surveys to define success and develop and stick to timelines *(WHO/ UNICEF, 2005)*.

Over the past 10 years, progress has been made in both water and sanitation. Focusing on Africa, Asia, Latin America and the Caribbean, it is clear that small changes have occurred and in the right direction *(Figure 3.4)* *(WHO/UNICEF, 2002)*. Yet, the

FIGURE 3.4

Geographic Population Without Safe Water and Sanitation

		YEAR	WATER	SANITATION
	Africa	1990	41%	41%
		2000	36%	40%
Source: WHO/ UNICEF Joint Monitoring Programme, 2002.	Asia	1990	27%	71%
		2000	19%	53%
	Latin America/ Caribbean	1990	18%	28%
		2000	13%	22%

remaining unserved populations are remarkable *(Figure 3.5)*. Geography makes a difference as well when you compare rural and urban areas. Overall, urban populations will continue to grow through 2025, while rural populations remain relatively flat. As for the unserved portion of the population, projections suggest urban areas will outperform rural, and water provision will outperform

FIGURE 3.5

2002 Unserved Individuals

	WATER	SANITATION
Global Total	**18%** (1.1 billion)	**42%** (2.6 billion)
Asia	65%	80%
Africa	27%	13%
Latin America/ Caribbean	6%	5%
Europe	2%	2%
Total	100%	100%

Source: UN Water for Life Decade WHO/UNICEF, 2002.

the extension of sanitation facilities. In general, the pace of prog ress will need to quicken in these areas to keep in step with health needs and population growth. Sanitation progress will lag behind in part because it "suffers from lack of natural demand." Compared with fresh water, the poor can more easily survive without sophis- ticated piped sewage systems which require high investment. Yet, as we've seen, absent good hygiene practices and sanitation, the water you get may not be clean.

Developed nations are not without water and sanitation health risk. All one need do is scan the local news to detect regular out- breaks of bacterial or parasitic infections, high mercury or lead levels in fish or drinking water or outbreaks of red tide affecting shellfish. Some crises are related to system contamination of piped water or non-point-of-source urban or agricultural runoff (EPA, 2005). Others are caused by careless food preparation. Others are the result of contaminated food imports and manufacturing prac- tices. Hurricane Katrina in 2005 dramatically demonstrated that citizens of the developed world are just as vulnerable as those in developing nations in the face of poor water disaster preparedness. So even for our human populations who are adequately resourced, water consumption and contamination both from the standpoint of quantity and quality and careful disaster preparedness and management must be carefully monitored literally on a day to day basis.

Today our human population finds itself in a different place than in 1970. At that time, the focus was on affirming our human population's basic needs, and of course water was at the top of the list. By the 1990s the notion of sustainable development took hold and wise management of water was clearly viewed as essential for the attainment of a wide range of social goals, from eliminating poverty to maintaining peace and security. Now Integrated Water Resource Management (IWRM) is front and center — the "multiple health dimensions of water for people, for food, for the environment." Suddenly water and sanitation are not standalones, but part of a broad development plan inclusive of the fight against poverty and the challenge of economic development. In philosophic terms, the WHO Committee on Economic, Social and Cultural Rights in 2000 put it this way, "Water is fundamental for a life of human dignity. It is a prerequisite to the realization of all other human rights."

The right to water then is the right to health. How best to implement that right is now up for debate. Certainly the need for integration is broadly accepted. Decentralization of planning and efficient execution are also on the rise. The advantages: creation of programs and priorities that consider local need, community mobilization and local maintenance and quality control. The challenges: building adequate capacity, overcoming local resistance and addressing a resource decision-making process which is still highly centralized. The loss of centralization also spells the loss of reliable epidemiologic surveillance, reliable monitoring and crisis response. Knowledge of the links between water and sanitation cause and disease effect can be difficult to access locally. On the other hand, done well, knowledge can accumulate locally and solutions can be customized. In fact, we are learning that "major health gains can be achieved at the household level through personal protection." Communities of health workers, sanitation engineers and environmental inspectors, each with a water role, may more easily interface on a local level, with their community at stake, than on a national level.

Still, there remain two critical points of focus that require a high level of empowerment if global health objectives are to be achieved. First, "keeping pace with a net population growth" means investing more and applying it more wisely and efficiently in the next decade. Second, we must recognize that sanitation lags behind water—and without good sanitation, long term, we can not ensure that the water we do have will be reliably clean and safe.

A river seems a magic thing.

A magic, moving, living part of the very earth itself —

for it is from the soil, both from its depth

and from its surface, that a river has its beginning.

— Laura Gilpin

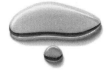

CHAPTER 4 **Water and Agriculture**

When it comes to water consumption, humans don't even come close to plants. Up to 70% of the water we extract from surface and ground water reserves goes to agriculture. Over the past few decades, food production has grown in tandem with population growth. But each year we come up short with some 800 million undernourished worldwide; and pockets of famine and human misery, complicated by natural and man-made disasters, remain relatively commonplace *(UN, 2003)*.

On a worldwide scale, agriculture has been a remarkable success story, keeping general pace with a human population that has roughly doubled in the last half century. In this context, the term agriculture is used to refer to plant growth, livestock husbandry, managed fisheries and forestry. How have they done it? They've done it with new high-yielding seeds, new plants, better central strategies — but most of all, with water. Population drives food, and food drives water. The problem is this: over the next 25 years, it is expected that developing countries will increase water withdrawal for agriculture by 14%, but efficient use of water will improve by only 4%. This negative balance, unaddressed, ensures non-sustainability *(FAO, 2002)*.

Worldwide expansion of irrigated land is projected to grow 23% in the next 25 years. Not all the water directed toward food will actually get there. Some leaks away by defective delivery, much evaporates and some feeds weeds. Dollars invested in irrigation roughly track food prices around the world. Early investment in irrigation has paid off in productivity, and price for food has declined. Many of the original irrigation programs were large public works. The transferability of these efforts is now under consideration, and the impact of large-scale irrigation farming on other issues of sustainability is being more carefully assessed.

As the world entered the new Millennium, the challenge was reflected in the numbers. 75% of the world's undernourished people as of 1999 were located in just 10 nations: India, China, Bangladesh, Democratic Republic of the Congo, Ethiopia, Pakistan, Philippines, Brazil, Tanzania and Vietnam. More remarkable: 48% resided in just two nations, India and China *(Figure 4.1)*. In terms of

FIGURE 4.1

Top Ten Undernourished Populations
(in millions)

533 MILLION
(75% of Global Total)

48% of Global Total	India	225
	China	116
	Bangladesh	44
	Democratic Republic of the Congo	31
	Ethiopia	30
	Pakistan	24
	Philippines	17
	Brazil	16
	Tanzania	16
	Vietnam	14

Source: FAO, 2002.

percentage of population, 10 nations have more than 45% of their population who are undernourished, including Somalia, Burundi, Democratic Republic of the Congo, Afghanistan, Eritrea, Haiti, Mozambique, Angola, Ethiopia and Kenya *(Figure 4.2) (FAO, 2000, 2001, 2002)*.

Calorie consumption varies from nation to nation. If one looks at per capita caloric intake in developed industrialized countries,

FIGURE 4.2

**Countries with More Than 45%
Undernourished Population (1999)**

Somalia	**75%**
Burundi	**66%**
Democratic Republic of the Congo	**64%**
Afghanistan	**58%**
Eritrea	**57%**
Haiti	**56%**
Mozambique	**54%**
Angola	**51%**
Ethiopia	**49%**
Kenya	**46%**

Source: FAO, 2000, 2001, 2002.

developing countries and those in transition, as of 1990, developed countries' per capita intake exceeded transition countries by 14% and developing countries by 21% *(Figure 4.3)*. Projections in each

FIGURE 4.3

**Calorie Consumption:
Narrowing the Gap Between
Developed and Developing**
(per capita per day)

	1998	PROJECTED 2015	PROJECTED 2030	PROJECTED INCREASE
Developed Countries (industrialized)	**3,380**	**3,440**	**3,500**	**+3.5%**
Transition Countries	**2,906**	**3,060**	**3,180**	**+9.4%**
Percentage Less Than Developed Countries	**−14%**	**−11%**	**−9%**	
Developing Countries	**2,681**	**2,850**	**2,980**	**+11.2%**
Percentage Less Than Developed Countries	**−21%**	**−17%**	**−15%**	

Source: FAO, 2002.

group of nations predict growth of 3.5% by 2030 for developed nations, 9.4% for transition countries and 11.2% for developing countries. If projections hold up, per capita caloric intake as of 2030 in developed nations will continue to exceed developing nations by 520 calories or 17% *(FAO, 2002)*.

What people eat changes as they eat more. This is the result of markets which reflect both preferences in food and access to preferred foods. Agriculture, in its planting choices, feeds the markets. Were agriculture to develop naturally, without markets defining prices and supporting farmers' labor and land use, it is estimated that natural output of plant growth would be only 10% of current yield with capacity to feed only 600 million rather than 6 billion *(Mazoyer and Roudart, 1998)*. Another way of saying it is that 90% of our world's population would be at risk without the orchestrated deliverable efforts of farmers, small and large, industrial and family, worldwide. But many indigenous people continue to subsist on natural food systems — fishing, gathering, hunting — under the radar screen of monitoring systems.

The bulk of managed agriculture is directed at grain cereals *(Figure 4.4) (FAO, 2002)*. The annual world production of cereals grew from just 1 billion tons in 1965 to 1.89 billion tons (+89%)

FIGURE 4.4

Annual World Production of Cereals

YEAR	GLOBAL PRODUCTION	INCREASE
1965	1 billion tons	—
1998	1.89 billion tons	+89%
Projected 2020	2.8 billion tons	+180%

Source: FAO, 2002.

Between 1962 and 1996, the amount of land required to grow the same amount of grain decreased by 56%.

by 1998. Growth over the next two decades is expected to rise to 2.8 billion tons (+180%). Not all is produced on-site. For example, cereal imports in the developing countries grew from 39 to 103 million tons between 1975 and 1998. Not all of these cereals go to humans. Approximately 44% are used to feed livestock, and 5% used for industrial use or waste. That leaves roughly 50% of all cereal crops for humans. These crops have been especially critical in the developing world, where cereal consumption in 1970 was 41 kilograms per person per year, and in 2000 had risen to 73 kilograms per person per year (56% of total calories). A decline in cereal's percentage of diet is occurring in both developing and developed nations, as diets diversify with nutritional advances. 20% of added calories in developing countries have come from food oil, including palm, soy, sunflower, sesame and coconut. Demand for food oil crops not only comes from human consumption but also from livestock and industrial use. Overall, however, for the foreseeable future, cereals will be the mainstay of human food consumption, and therefore will be well-represented in expenditure of agricultural resources *(FAO, 2000, 2001)*.

As populations increase, food production will likely grow as well. This can be accomplished by expanding the amount of land in use, expanding the number of crops and shortening the time to maturity and expanding yield per acre. In the past 50 years, agricultural land use has increased 12%, so that today 11% of all of the planet's land surface is committed to agriculture. Yet, when measured against population growth, planted land per person has actually declined 40%, reflecting increased efficiencies and decreased costs. Yield in tons of crop doubled from 1962 to 1996. The amount of land required to deliver a fixed amount of grain declined by 56%. For the developing world, future agricultural growth will come primarily from efficiencies (80%) and only secondarily from expanded land use (20%). Developing countries will increase land use by approximately 13% in the next 25 years, mainly in sub-Saharan Africa and

Latin America. As diets in developing countries have evolved, livestock has become increasingly important. Growing at a rate of 5% to 6% a year, markets now aggressively support beef, pork, poultry, eggs and dairy products. Poultry growth has been especially vibrant, more than doubling from 13% to 28% of meat output worldwide in the past 50 years. This reflects growth in protein consumption as living conditions have risen *(UN, 2003)*.

As meat consumption has risen so has annual fish consumption, reaching 16.3 kg per capita in 1999, and expected to increase an additional 23% by 2030. This will translate into over 150 million tons of fish produced, up from 130 million tons currently. Of this, three-quarters is consumed by humans. The other quarter, in the form of fish meal and fish oil, is consumed as food by other fish or livestock. 27% of current fish production comes from aquaculture and 73% from marine and inland capture. Of the latter—some 85 million tons per year — there remains marginal growth potential, since drawing beyond 100 million tons per year from oceans and rivers, it is believed, would threaten the base of these species. The future, then, is in aquaculture, which has been growing at an annual clip of 10% through the 1990s. Of the 35 million tons of aquaculture fish currently harvested, 40% is marine-based and 60% from inland waters. Developing countries have led the way, controlling 90% of aquaculture, 70% alone coming from China *(Figure 4.5) (UNEP, 2002)*. Success brings additional challenges, such as understanding environmental impacts and ecosystem management of these highly profitable ventures which now exceed earnings from traditional crops like coffee and bananas. Issues such as fish farm waste, chemical and drug pollution, transference of disease and parasites from escape of farm fish into the wild and drawing down of wild fish supplies in order to provide feed for farmed fish (it takes 3 pounds of wild fish to produce 1 pound of farmed salmon) are now surfacing for debate *(UN, 2003; FAO, 2000)*.

In general, as populations in developing countries grow, dependence on agriculture will continue to rise. While aquaculture fish crops

FIGURE 4.5

Growth in Aquaculture

Growth:	• Aquaculture supply doubled between 1984 and 1994.
Output:	• Aquaculture produces 27% of all fish consumed globally.
Source:	• 70% of the total aquaculture "crop" comes from China.
Future:	• Fish consumption is expected to increase 23% between 2002 and 2030.

Source: UNEP, 2002.

are a growing export, cereals will continue to be an important import, especially in the developing world where the land often cannot meet the needs. Part of the reason is that water, in various areas, is not sufficient to support direct and indirect human needs. Water for drinking must trump water for agriculture. So, net imports of cereals in developing countries will rise to just under 200 million tons by 2015, and will increase an additional 33% by 2030. Imports of cereals in general do not exceed 20% of total demand. That said, for countries with true water scarcity, it is less expensive to import water as food in its original form. Food in this case is "virtual water." A unit of cereal consumes 1.5 units of water. The ratios for poultry and beef are 6 to 1, and 15 to 1 respectively *(Figure 4.6) (FAO, 1997; UN, 2003)*.

In the developing world, 60% of agricultural production is rainfed, and therefore variable. Careful soil planning can direct runoff to roots and improve ground water recharging. But the absence of irrigation greatly increases the chance of total crop loss, and therefore restricts willingness of farmers to invest in equipment or newer soil additives whether they be high-yield seeds, nutrients or pesticides that would lead to predictably higher yields were water to be ensured. Even if seasonal rains deliver the same quantity, albeit erratically, as irrigation, in a single season, studies show that natural agriculture

FIGURE 4.6

"Virtual Water":
Water Is Food, Food Is Water
(volume [cubic meters])

WATER REQUIRED TO PRODUCE
(1 kg)

Citrus Fruit	**1.0m³**
Cereal	**1.5m³**
Palm Oil	**2.0m³**
Chicken	**6.0m³**
Lamb	**10.0m³**
Beef	**15.0m³**

Source: FAO, 1997.

yields reach only 43% of those derived from high-input irrigated crops. While only one-fifth of developing world agriculture utilizes irrigation, it produces up to three-fifths of their cereal agricultural output. Irrigated fields have a 400% greater grain output than refined fields *(FAO, 2001; UN, 2003)*.

Irrigation of lands in developing countries is expected to grow an additional 20% by 2030, but overall rates of increase in irrigation worldwide are slowing down. The net increase between now and 2030 will be less than half the rate of increase in the prior 36 years. This reflects lower projected growth in food demands, rising cost of irrigation and competition for land from industry and urban growth as economies advance. Growth, then, in irrigation will primarily be in converting existing rain-fed fields rather than accessing new land, especially in Asia, North Africa and the Middle East. But water extracted is not the same as water delivered to the roots of plants. In general, only 38% of water extracted in the developing world for irrigation reaches its target *(UN, 2003)*. By 2030, predicted delivery percentages vary from lows in Latin America and sub-Saharan Africa of 25% and 37%, to highs in North Africa and South Asia of 53% and 49% *(FAO, 2002)*.

While total land use for irrigated agriculture is relatively small, water consumed is not. Of the 93 developing nations recently surveyed, 10 were consuming more than 10% of their renewable water for this purpose. By 2030, South Asia and North Africa will be consuming 41% and 58% of their renewable water to irrigate their fields. Increasingly farmers have turned to ground water, which is available and on time. It also is under the farmers' rather than the government's control. Drawbacks are obvious, notably declining water levels. Near the sea, over-pumping of aquifers often leads to increased salinity, which may occur slowly but has a lasting effect (FAO, 2002).

Natural aquifers do not suffer the same climate-driven variations as exposed surface water. Of course, accessing ground water requires pumping, which requires investment. If thoroughly subsidized, there may be little incentive for the farmer to carefully manage what is in fact a very valuable and potentially limited commodity. As water is drawn off, pumps must go deeper. Deeper pumps cost more, causing poorer farmers to drop out first. In addition, some of the aquifers are contained in relatively impenetrable fossil rock containers, and are therefore less renewable. Such is the case in both the Middle East and North Africa. In Saudi Arabia, more water is currently drawn from aquifers than is annually renewable (UN, 2003).

Global agriculture capacity is judged adequate to feed our growing worldwide populations for at least the next 25 years. But the reality is that the food is not equitably distributed. 1998 figures showed 815 million undernourished people, with 95% in developing countries, 3.5% in transition countries and 1.5% in developed countries. Shortages of food in some areas are chronic, while in others are stimulated by man made or natural disasters. The focus of worldwide aid agencies is on stabilizing vulnerable populations and raising their strength and health back to baseline levels so that, with guidance and investment, they might move to a more secure and sustainable nutritional baseline.

It is important to remember that water confers multiple advantages to at-risk populations. Not only does it ensure greater quantity, quality and diversity of food, but also it provides direct income and employment to large portions of the population. Indirect income generation reaches an even wider population involved with sale of equipment, seed, nutrients and fertilizer, or participating in the sale and distribution of local food. Where land is irrigated in India, fewer than three in 10 live in poverty. Where it is not, seven in 10 live in poverty *(World Bank, 1991)*. In many areas, irrigation is local and small-scale, involving modest ground water pumping from shallow aquifers. Community support and planning can stabilize small, rural populations. Produce can be sold locally, providing income. In some of the larger and more organized sites, there may be traditional access to credit and insurance against crop failure. But in most areas, "non-conventional credit systems"— or neighbors covering each other's needs, building trust equity and accomplishing solidarity —help to stabilize a community.

In other areas, with differing geology and access to financial resources, projects take on a decidedly larger scale. Libya is such an example. Largely desert surveys revealed some 120,000 cubic kilometers of fresh water, hidden and undisturbed for likely 40,000 years deep beneath the sand. Twenty years after construction began, 6 million cubic meters of water flow across the Sahara to population centers and fields, accessed through nearly 400 miles of pipe that are connected to the ancient water source *(UN, 2003)*.

Some large-scale projects involve not only significant engineering but also great social complexity. The Senegal River basin is an example. In the lower valley area, annual rainfall is nearly always limited. Food production has been traditionally marginal and, at times of drought, can catastrophically fail. In 1972, the Organization for the Development of the Senegal River was formed. Over the past 30 years, dams have been built, irrigated land extended, crops mixed and diversified, pasture and wooded area for nearly 3 million cattle and 4.5 million sheep and goats secured and fishing yield between 25 and 50 thousand tons maintained. The effort on one level requires access to financial, governmental and technical resources. On another level, it is a most complex societal effort integrating water maintenance and economy with agriculture, animal husbandry, forestry and fishing. Increasingly fish are a sizable protein source and economic stabilizer within local markets. Increasing success in fishing not only is evident in Asia but also sub-Saharan Africa, including stocking efforts for natural and man-made bodies of water and aquaculture techniques. Beyond the traditional nutritional benefits, direct benefits to health occur. For example, rice fields often breed malaria-containing mosquitoes. By raising fish and rice side by side, both cereal and proteins are created, and fish consume mosquito larvae with resultant declines in malaria among the population (UN, 2003).

While water access and food security are obviously linked, proximity does not ensure success. In fact, much of the governmental investment of the 1960s and 1970s fell short of its goals either by poor design, follow-through or maintenance. By the 1980s, investment had dropped by 50%, with further declines in the 1990s. As investment was going down, cost of irrigation programs was going up, in some cases by as much as 50% (UN, 2003). These realities are stimulating significant rethinking of how best to invest in water-driven, agricultural progress. For one thing, private investment is growing and now represents approximately 15% of available irrigation system development currency. Responsibility is increasingly being placed on the shoulders of local farmers for both operation and maintenance. Water-use associations are being established early. Supply orientation is gradually giving way to service orientation, which implies changes in planning, technology, measurement and continuous improvement. In general, control of governmental-held systems is slowly being transferred to water-use associations and service-providing companies. Such a transition is neither smooth nor uncomplicated. It is not easy to remove political influence or adequately involve poor stakeholders. Costs can rise as numbers of stakeholders involved increase. Adequately distributing risk and benefit across the new governing entity and the various populations served can be enormously controversial. For example, breaking through gender bias is not easy. Not only are women major transporters and users of water, in some studies they appear to be better irrigation farmers. So in some areas, small plots are now designated separately to men and women rather than just routinely transferred to head of household *(UN, 2003)*.

More productivity is not simply more food. One must assess the overall benefits and risks. One must consider the negatives as well as positives. That agriculture is a major consumer of the Earth's natural resources is undeniable. Currently agriculture utilizes 37% of the Earth's land surface. It accounts for approximately 70% of all human consumption of water. It is the main source of nitrate and ammonia pollution of surface water and aquifers. It delivers phosphates into our water, and methane and nitrous oxides into our air. Poorly conceived efforts to improve agriculture can have devastating and lasting impact. Take, for example, the Aral Sea debacle. In the 1950s Khrushchev diverted two Russian rivers to supply profitable cotton fields in the region. Using open ditch irrigation, 80% of the water was lost to evaporation and seepage. Over the next few decades, the Aral Sea shrunk to half its size, salinity rose and fish died. Sixty thousand residents living off the sea were impacted immediately. With the passage of time, dust from the sea's contaminated seabed, picked up by winds, spread across the Antarctic, and deposited on Himalayan peaks where the salt caused early melting of snow. One ill-advised policy choice created a lasting impact around the world *(Health Politics, 2004)*.

Clearly, sound planning and decision making will become increasingly critical as populations rise and water becomes more scarce. Good decision making can turn a liability into an opportunity. For example, poorly planned, agriculture's extension into wetlands can eliminate a strategic ecologic, botanical and zoologic resource, impacting both biodiversity and protective flood plains. But if one selects the right crops, manages water and has a well-thought-out watershed plan, dual use may be appropriate and beneficial in certain areas.

In looking ahead, it is likely that agriculture will continue to be our dominant consumer of water for the foreseeable future. It is also likely that, done well, and integrated with other community priorities, irrigation has the ability to expand yield and improve the economies of developing and transition nations by impacting plant, fish and meat yields. At the same time, the critical nature of food security, transitional forms of public and private water planning and governments and large-scale agriculture's and aquaculture's capacity to create wide-scale negative environment impacts all speak to the need for wise, integrated planning. Our food supplies are more than adequate, though they continue to suffer by distribution. Our water supplies are today more stressed, and ill-distributed. What all must realize is that you cannot manage one without managing the other. Food is water, and water is food.

Let there be work, bread, water and salt for all.

— *Nelson Mandela*

CHAPTER 5 # Water and Industry

It is only a trick of the human mind that could allow us to think of water and industry as disconnected. On the one hand, there is scarcely a product produced by industry that doesn't either incorporate water in its construction, to cool or heat engines, to cleanse or deliver materials. On the other hand, it is from industry that we derive a wide range of products that allow humans to access, cleanse, transport and deliver water.

Water and industry have grown up side by side, broadly advancing economic and social progress, aiding in creation of products and then transporting these products over waterways to sites far and wide. In our modern world, we are witnessing export of industrial capacity to the developing world on a large scale to achieve a comparative cost advantage. Such transfers carry many advantages for local populations. But less visible is the additional burden on already stressed water supplies.

Not only may quantity of water be impacted, but also quality. From a quantity perspective, industry is not nearly the consumer of energy that agriculture is, being responsible for roughly 22% of water use worldwide versus 70% for agriculture *(World Bank, 2001)*. Its lower use is a reflection of the fact that industry only infrequently consumes or permanently extracts water from the system. Most of the water used is not incorporated into product, but utilized indirectly and then returned as wastewater into sewage systems or directly into a waterway.

Industry requires quality water for most manufacturing, but may return water in a degraded state at the other end of the process. The volume of water can be considerable. So while not consumed in quantity, industry can alter large volumes of water; and if directly discharged into waterways, this water can have a significant negative health impact on surface and ground reserves. If discharged into sewage lines, the clean-up often falls on governmental treatment plants, and becomes a cost of development versus a cost to industry, where the water degradation occurred.

The amount of water accessed by industry varies widely by geography. In 2001, higher income countries' industry used 59% of the water, while agriculture consumed just 30%, with 11% going to domestic uses. In middle-income countries, industry consumed 13%, agriculture 74% and domestic 12%. In lower income countries, just 8% was industrial, 87% agricultural and 5% domestic. Even within this last category, certain sub-areas were outliers. For example, South Asia utilized just 2% of its water in association with industry, 93% for agriculture and just 4% for domestic use *(Figure 5.1) (World Bank, 2001).*

FIGURE 5.1

2001 Water Usage

		AGRICULTURE	INDUSTRY	DOMESTIC
	High-Income Nations	30%	59%	11%
	Middle-Income Nations	74%	13%	12%
Source: World Bank, 2001.	Low-Income Nations	87%	8%	5%

A wide range of financial incentives as well as contractual arrangements have begun to shape the amount of water supplied, and industries' demand for that water. There has been movement toward front-end consideration of economic versus environmental objectives and incentives. Consideration of investment in new technologies as well as processes internally that could increase water efficiency and decrease demand are now more frequently brought into play. Advanced planning also provides the opportunity to consider pollutant loads and alternate discharge routes, either by capture or reuse of excess raw materials.

Emissions of organic water pollutants vary by industry. Those industries with an organic product lead the pack. In low-income countries, the food and beverage industries generate 54% of organic pollution, followed by textiles (15%), paper and pulp (10%), chemicals (7%), metal (7%) and wood (5%) *(World Bank, 2001)*. Around the globe, industries are usually established near human settlements. This provides a workforce whose local communities could be enhanced by strong health advocacy and an improved infrastructure with the potential to challenge poor practices with well-thought-out reforms.

More developed nations are further along in the planning process. Such planning considers conflicting needs and demands for resources. Abstractions of water are more strictly controlled and water is fully valued economically. Often, to be licensed, one must demonstrate a plan to maximize, sustain and protect natural resources. Thus industrial progress in developed countries has driven water savings in response to governmentally mandated integrated water management. They then have transferred a portion of the knowledge and industrial capacity to their plants in the developing world.

Where industries tended to grow up around water-based communities in the developed nations, many of the new manufacturing sites in impoverished markets are situated not to advantage water but rather to access lower labor costs, tax advantages and ease of export shipment. Responsibility for water development often exists in a different silo than industrial development. So industry comes in without full local understanding of its water impact, and then delivers a secondary blow by instigating local urbanization with increased domestic water consumption, as the workforce follows the jobs.

A portion of the new industries still seek water sites, especially on rivers. The rivers generally cross national boundaries. Lack of regulations on contaminants and pollutant loads upstream impacts resources downstream. Lack of dedicated or underpowered municipal treatment facilities are frequently a source of problems. Such issues, understood and properly addressed, can yield long-term benefits. In January 2000, a dam on the Szamos River in Romania released tons of cyanide-contaminated sludge into the Szamos and Tisza Rivers, and from there to the Danube and Black Sea, with both human and environmental impacts. In response, the United Nations Industrial Development Organization (UNIDO) initiated a pilot project that began with a formal risk assessment, addressed gaps in early monitoring, developed preventive measures, improved cross-sector communication, developed emergency response preparedness and developed long-term leadership and policy recommendations *(EEC, 2000)*.

Addressing knowledge gaps can yield significant improvements. Clearly, in some cases, leaders' desire for improved economic performance makes them reluctant to balance long-term resource needs against industry short-term success. At other times, problems arise from the use of inefficient or inappropriate technologies or from lack of technical expertise in the enterprise. Managers may be fundamentally unaware how water is being used and for what purpose. Measurement of consumption may not be part of the process at all, so management becomes inconsequential. Improving skill levels and education regarding the joint economic and environmental advantages of process re-engineering and incorporation of modern technologies may have a greater impact directed at owners and workers than at public officials. Wasting raw materials is, after all, a waste. Why throw out dyes used for textiles if you can recapture them. And along the way, you can reduce oxygen demand of the water.

One area of growing concern is the location of industry in coastal zones. Such zones are especially vulnerable since they are the receiving points of converging river basins, and are at the interface of sea and fresh water. UNIDO has embraced dealing with the pollutants at sources upstream as the best strategy for control. But there are a wide range of local coastal issues beyond toxic discharge, including over-fishing, sediment flow from land mismanagement, coral mining, canalizing wetlands, aquifer salination and sand filling to name a few. Coastal governance is complex. On-site fishery ministries, tourism ministries and environmental ministries are driven by different priorities and agendas. Inland sprawl seems a world apart from coastal wetlands, and jurisdictional disputes are commonplace *(UNIDO, 2001)*.

Traditional concepts, such as polluter pays, seem reasonable — but the reality is that they only act where pollution is obvious and provable, resolution is often long delayed, cross-jurisdiction feuding is common, technical assistance is often lacking and legal access to involved parties may be obstructed. For these reasons and more, proper planning and positive engagement of industry, with a focus on quantity of water used, quality of water returned and overall corporate citizenship and involvement in integrated water management plans, are increasingly embraced. The goal? According to UNIDO, "consensus between community, industry and government actors, early in planning and investment processes. Within industry, a progressive package of environmentally-sensitive improvements needs to be incorporated into production management and combined with the raising of technical capabilities at all levels" *(UN, 2003; UNIDO, 2002)*.

When approached this way, UNIDO has documented significant progress. For example, they have worked with 30 tanneries in nine African nations since 1988 on waste management and cleaner leather-making technologies. One action, the use of high exhaustion chrome tanning technology, reduced the amount of chrome in effluent by 90% and covered costs since less chrome was required to create product. Another experiment with the Zimbabwe Bata Shoe Company used an anaerobic digester of sludge, converting the output to zero solid waste and creating an energy source in the process.

Work with the Thien Huong Food Company in Vietnam resulted in 62 cleaner production options, with 24 put into practice. One year later, wastewater release was down 68% and organic waste output down 35%. Every dollar invested saved 10 dollars in production. Positive collaboration aims then at decreases in industry emissions, more efficient production and better product quality *(UN, 2003)*.

What of the future? Needs for water and industry are now better defined. We need verifiable statistics, more reliable consumption indicators, improved industrial efficiency, water re-use, recycling indicators, water quality measures and implementation of smartest technology. On the regional level, we need better, more representative governance, multinational river basin and trans-boundary agreements, acceptance of water management by industry as a priority, proactive definition of risk and threats and emphasis on sustainability. And locally, we need engagement of industry in economics and environment, voluntary consensus, careful data collection and clean, efficient production.

All water has a perfect memory and is forever

 trying to get back to where it was.

 — *Toni Morrison*

CHAPTER 6 Water and Energy

As we have seen, for the human race to reach its full potential, and to secure a sustainable future, we need water, food and industrial production. What we have not yet acknowledged is that, except for a relatively small percentage, we could not have any of the above without energy.

All the more striking then that 2 billion of Earth's inhabitants have no energy at all, and an additional 1 billion rely on batteries, candles and kerosene *(UNDP, 2004)*. Three million use biomass fuel and coal for cooking and home heating. With this type of need, it is not surprising that demand for electricity is growing, and that consumption is expected to increase some 15% in the next 20 years. Developed countries are currently accessing only 70% of their true electricity potential, while developing nations are utilizing only 15% of their potential *(UN, 2003)*. Lack of energy in the developing world is just one more obstacle to breaking out of poverty. Beyond higher costs, absent or restricted energy means women are burdened with fetching water and gathering wood for fuel, employment opportunities are few and far between, educational facilities are unlit and low-tech, large-scale agriculture is undermined and health services in general are compromised. This multifaceted assault on basic needs is a reality in both urban and rural environments. As to what is the best source of energy, electricity is a clear winner, at least for lighting, generating 10 times the light at less than the cost of kerosene.

Electricity changes women's lives. From household duties to gathering fuel, the daily load is lighter. Managing chores and stress opens time for productive employment, for education, for relation-ship-building. Lighting in the evening permits learning. Micro-enterprises either consume fuel, as in cooking, or utilize lighting, as with home-based evening work. Without electricity, many ventures are no longer profitable or safe. Also, in the absence of electricity, low-efficiency biomass stores create an internal environment filled with carbon monoxide, carcinogens and particulate matter, which undermine family health.

From a pure health perspective, electricity is a life-enhancer. Food preparation is more secure and water can be boiled. Fires are less likely. Health facilities can refrigerate and sterilize and can operate at night. And health information and instructions can be mass-communicated. But in rural settings, cost/benefit weighs in. Except for lighting, you can accomplish domestic tasks less expen-sively with other fuels. Water can be hand-pumped. High efficiency stoves can use fossil fuels. However, as personal economy or expec-tations for improved standard of living through entrepreneurship arise, electricity becomes a critical lever. The challenge is to manage its distribution so as not to exacerbate existing disparities.

In the developing world, Africa lags considerably behind Asia, the Middle East, Latin America and the Caribbean in access to domestic electricity. As of 1995, the numbers were dramatic. Chad — 2.8% of households had electricity; Central African Republic — 5%; Uganda — 6.9%; Niger — 7.9%; Tanzania — 8.9%; Mozambique — 9.9%; Madagascar — 11.1%; Kenya — 11.7%; Nigeria — 25.5%. Of 22 African nations noted in the survey, only three approach access for one-third of their population. In Asia, only Nepal (18%) and Bangladesh (24.9%) are similarly deprived. India (51.5%) and Morocco (46.9%) fall in a mid-range, while the remaining eight nations noted range from 63% to 100%. In Latin America and the Caribbean, Haiti is an outlier at 31%, Paraguay (49.2%) and Gua-temala (58.7%) in mid-range, with the remaining six between 67% and 93%. In all areas, access to electricity tracks with income levels, with the poor severely impacted *(Water Power and Dam Construction, 1995; Danis, 1995)*.

In rural areas, 85% of energy is consumed by homes, primarily for cooking and heating. Agriculture consumes only about 5%. Commercial energy, mainly for lighting, accounts for less than 10% of use in village enterprises *(UN, 2003)*. As means rise, better lighting is a top priority. With it comes extension of the workday and enhancements in productivity. As means rise further, the comparative luxuries of refrigeration and cooling are fueled.

As integrated planning for sustainable development has expanded, priorities are weighed, often one against the other. Water and energy intersect dramatically in the area of hydropower. Underutilized, accessible, clean and relatively well-distributed, hydropower holds significant promise. As of 2001, hydropower provided 19% of the world's total electricity. 64% of global energy was thermal, and 17% was nuclear *(Figure 6.1) (IHA, 2002)*. Of total potential hydropower

FIGURE 6.1

2002 Global Energy Sources

	Thermal	**64%**
	Hydro	**19%**
Source: IHA, 2002.	Nuclear	**17%**

resources, 26% is currently in place, 3% under construction and 71% still to be built and placed on-line. Of the existing capacity, some 94% is derived from large hydroelectric projects, while 6% comes from small local access projects. Hydropower currently supplies 50% of electrical production in 66 countries and at least 90% in 24 countries *(UN, 2003)*.

Approximately half of all water power comes from Europe and North America. The United States is the second largest producer of hydroelectric, where it accounts for 12% of total electric production. Hydropower is projected to increase worldwide by 77% when one

FIGURE 6.2

**Projected Hydropower Growth
(1995–2010)**
(Terawatt hours per year)

	1995	PROJECTED 2010	GROWTH
Worldwide	2,380	4,210	+77%
NAFTA Nations	653	710	+9%
Latin America	465	1,000	+115%
European Union	441	493	+12%
Asia	333	1,100	+230%
Former USSR	160	400	+150%
Australia/ Japan/ New Zealand	132	141	+7%
Africa	67	150	+24%
Central/ Eastern Asia	62	99	+60%
Turkey/Cyprus/ Gibraltar/Malta	36	73	+28%
Middle East	25	50	+100%

Source:
International
Journal on
Hydropower
and Dams, 1997.

compares 1995 levels with estimated 2010 levels *(Figure 6.2) (International Journal on Hydropower and Dams, 1997)*. Hydropower is already the dominant power source in many developing nations as well, including Afghanistan, Congo, Ethiopia, Mozambique, Nepal, Rwanda, Sri Lanka, Uganda and Zaire. China's investment in hydroelectric is unparalleled. Hydroelectric projects currently in construction, including the Three Gorges Dam, will produce 50 gigawatts of electricity, doubling the country's current capacity. An additional 28 gigawatts of construction are about to begin, with 80 gigawatts of hydro projects in the planning stages. In addition, China has some 60,000 small (less than 1 megawatt) hydroelectric schemes *(UN, 2003)*.

Hydroelectric is a critical element in the campaign to control global warming from greenhouse gases. Every additional terawatt of hydropower per hour, in displacing coal-generated electricity, eliminates 1 million tons of carbon dioxide (CO_2) emitted into the atmosphere. As of 1995, human activities were generating some 23 billion tons of CO_2 a year, one third of which was produced by combustion of coal, oil and gas *(Water Power and Dam Construction, 1995)*.

In our modern world, hydroelectric has a great deal to offer. It's efficient and environmentally sensitive. It is sustainable in rural and urban settings. It emits no greenhouse gases, wastes or air pollutants. It is renewable, efficient, flexible, uses existing technology, is low maintenance and decreases pollutants from fossil fuel. These advantages need to be weighed against disadvantages, including high initial cost, impact on habitats, potential disturbance of water quality and forced migration of local populations *(Figure 6.3)*. In

FIGURE 6.3

Hydropower Highlights

Production:
· Hydropower generates 19% of global energy.
Prevalence: · 50% of countries have hydropower projects in process.
Use: · Hydropower produces the majority of energy for 66 nations.
Benefits: · Hydropower is renewable, economically viable and decreases greenhouse gases.
Concerns: · Hydropower requires dams, alters the environment and displaces species and human populations.

Source: UNEP, 2000.

addition, for large projects, one must add in the cost of connecting to the electric grid. Large scale and centrally managed grid options can prove a failure economically and ecologically *(UNEP, 2000)*. Much has been learned however from these failures, and there now exists a World Commission on Dams which is a unique consultative, planning, construction and management resource. Small scale, environmentally sound, off-grid hydropower schemes are also increasingly popular. These efforts capture the mechanical energy from water movement and convert it to electrical energy. The components include a reservoir, hydraulic controlled outlet, water channel directing flow to a turbine, power generation equipment and an exit channel to reunite water to a natural catchbasin.

Mini- and micro-hydropower projects avoid large dams, do not displace large populations and deliver electricity locally. Though small, the positive impacts can be considerable. A 1 megawatt plant will produce 6,000 megawatts of electricity for use by 1,500 families. To do the same with coal means dumping 4,000 tons of CO_2 and 275 tons of sulfur dioxide into the local environment *(UN, 2003)*. Most are "run of the river" schemes, which leave rivers intact and do not flood lands upstream or interfere with seasonal river flow downstream. There are no expensive flow controls. When the river is flowing, turbines operate and energy is produced. Construction of such a system is quite economical and usually managed using in-country expertise and readily available technology. One major negative is that such systems are decentralized and disconnected from each other and therefore resist distributive planning or movements toward economy of scale.

Where else might we find natural, sustainable energy? One obvious site is the ocean. Energy experts are developing approaches to capturing ocean energy in three differing forms: mechanical energy trapped in the tidal flow of water, wind energy trapped in the waves and thermal energy stored in warm surface waters. The Earth's surface as well may be a source of geothermal energy in the future, either through steam and hot water stores within the Earth or through geothermal heat pumps that take advantage of temperature differentials in the Earth.

So we see energy presents the human race with a wide variety of complex choices. To date we have largely fueled development with fossil fuel-generated energy. This choice over the past 100 years has sustained rapid growth and progress for a portion of our citizens. But 100 years is a very short time, and the negative impacts of this decision are already visible in the quality of our air, land and water. In fueling progress, we have created a CO_2 burden that is changing our weather patterns, and is difficult to reverse. Clearly, new energy solutions are in demand. And many energy experts around the world are looking to water for the answers.

The river moves from land to water to land,

in and out of organisms, reminding us

what native peoples have never forgotten:

that you cannot separate the land

from the water, or the people from the land.

— *Lynn Noel,* Voyages: Canada's Heritage Rivers

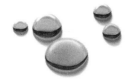

CHAPTER 7 Water
and
Cities

That cities will continue to grow into the future is not open for debate. People migrate towards population centers for jobs, for services, for opportunity, for a perceived better future. Whether their expectations are met is part personal initiative, part luck and part leadership. Leaders in these centers impact the urban economy, the politics, the social contracts, the educational opportunities, the health and, in sum, the life of new arrivals.

In the developing world, the history of urban populations is checkered at best. The WHO sees much of the infrastructure upon which services are based as less than adequate. Half the urban population is challenged with poor water or inadequate sanitation with resultant disease burden. 17% of the childhood population is dead before the age of five. In spite of this, cities continue to grow and, if managed well, provide advantages beyond those available in many rural settings *(WHO, 1999)*.

By 2030, 5 billion of the more than 8 billion global citizens will be urban dwellers *(Figure 7.1) (UNEP, 2002)*. In 1990, cities contained

FIGURE 7.1

Urban Population Growth

	YEAR	URBAN POPULATION	PERCENTAGE OF GLOBAL CITIZENS
	2000	**2 billion**	**43%**
	2004	**2.9 billion**	**46%**
	Projected 2025	**4 billion**	**60%**
Source: UNEP, 2002.	Projected 2030	**5 billion**	**63%**

only 15% of our population. By 2002, the number was 48%, and in 2030 it will be over 60%. Not only are overall numbers growing, but city size on average is expanding. The largest 100 cities in 1800 averaged a population of 200,000. One hundred years later, it was 700,000. But by 2000, 388 cities averaged 1 million plus inhabitants and 16% had more than 10 million, accounting for remarkable centralization of 4% of our entire global population. These cities are centered and fueled by Earth's largest regional economies. And they are also positioned in some of our most water-stressed geographic locations *(UN, 2002)*.

If you look at predicted movements of populations between 2000 and 2015, trends for both developed and developing nations show movement from rural to urban environments. For developed countries, urban residents will grow from 75% to 79% of the population, as rural populations decline from 25% to 21%. In developing nations, city residents will increase from 40% to 49% of the total population, and rural populations will decline from 60% to 51% of citizens *(Figure 7.2) (UNEP, 2002)*.

FIGURE 7.2

Population Distribution

			URBAN	RURAL
	Developed Countries	2000	75%	25%
		Projected 2015	79%	21%
	Developing Countries	2000	40%	60%
		Projected 2015	49%	51%
Source: UNEP, 2002.	Total	2000	47%	53%
		Projected 2015	54%	46%

The perceived benefits of this centralization of human capital in terms of opportunity rests heavily on both communal and domestic development, which translates quite directly into expanding demands for water. Not surprisingly then, most cities are progressively digging deeper for ground water and traveling farther to access surface water than ever before. Of the 2.9 billion current urbanites, some

60% are dependent on surface source water and 40% on ground source water. And they are not alone, but must compete with agricultural, industrial, energy and urban sprawl domestic consumers for an increasingly expensive resource. Yet those who have it are the lucky ones. For those who do not (some 6%), they generally must purchase vendor water at higher prices *(UN, 2003)*.

The world's 389 largest cities range from Tokyo, Japan with 26 million to Volgograd, Russia with 1 million citizens *(Figure 7.3)*

FIGURE 7.3

2002 Urban Populations

CITY	POPULATION (in millions)	GLOBAL RANK (in population)
Tokyo, Japan	26.4	1
London, UK	7.6	25
Milan, Italy	4.3	50
Recife, Brazil	3.4	75
Medellin, Columbia	2.9	100
Linyi, China	2.4	125
St. Louis, USA	2.0	150
Kyoto, Japan	1.9	175
Belem, Brazil	1.7	200
Pingxiang, China	1.5	225
Tbilisi, Georgia	1.4	250
Xintai, China	1.3	275
Hefei, China	1.2	300
Jingmen, China	1.2	325
Maputo, Mozambique	1.1	350
Chelyabinsk, Russia	1.0	375
Volgograd, Russia	1.0	389

Source: UN, 2002.

(UN, 2002). The history of urban water management is one of crisis and mismanagement, with leaders who seek the least expensive way to access and dispose of water. But over the course of years, the cost of failure, in dollars and political fallout, the rise of knowledge and expertise and the establishment of standards of measurement

and stable regulatory authorities have moved us at least in the right direction. But the truth remains that urban water and waste management, at best, is enormously complex. Water systems, waste systems, flood prevention, pollution management, sustainable resourcing while maintaining growth — all of this and more requires funding, planning, execution, monitoring and integration. It also requires standard setting, in that water supplied must be safe and affordable, and sanitation systems should be reliable, well-maintained and convenient.

Standards often must consider pragmatic realities. In more-developed countries, a standard that "all urban households have safe, regular piped water to their home, internal plumbing and their own sanitary toilet" is achievable. In a developing nation urban setting, pursuing this same standard might ensure ideal access to the richest 20% and no access at all to the poorest 80%. For such a circumstance, safe access to a tap within 50 meters of one's home that can provide a person with 20 liters of safe water per person per day may, more realistically, impact most of the population. Finally, one can build toward standards, but maintaining the infrastructure requires continued investment and improvements made reliably over time. Middle-income countries increasingly build toward higher standards but often underfund maintenance of the system. For lower income countries, efficiency, maintenance, pricing, supervision and regulation are the challenges. Their infrastructure is often incomplete, and management of what does exist remains highly variable. The populations come for better jobs and opportunities, but often inherit water that is heavily compromised by bacteria and pollutants (WHO, 2000).

On the other hand, cities have advantages when it comes to water. There exist economies of scale with larger enterprises that more easily support infrastructure investment. Average incomes are higher than for rural counterparts. People are concentrated, and therefore more easily within reach of mapped delivery systems for both water and sanitation. Done well and properly funded, urban migrants can expect major improvements in access to water and safe sanitation.

Done poorly, they can become entrapped in an explosive, disease-laden environment that can be life-threatening.

The presence of piped water, sanitation and garbage removal in a city directly impacts basic health. In well-developed cities, child mortality rates are commonly 10 per 100,000 live births. Where infrastructure is inadequate, child death rates are frequently increased by a factor of 10. And within the sub-segments of these cities, there exists great variability in a single city. A study of seven communities in Karachi, Pakistan, for example, revealed infant mortality rates from 33 to 209 per 100,000 live births. They die from water-borne cholera, typhoid, hepatitis B and even malaria, which has normally been a factor primarily in rural environments. They have worms, scabies and trachoma. They are malnourished, immune-depleted and in general vulnerable and at-risk *(Montgomery, 2002)*.

The extent of the urban challenges varies by geography. Of the 2.9 billion urban dwellers in 2002, 48% lived in Asia, 19% in Europe, 14% in Latin America and the Caribbean, 10% in Africa and 9% in North America *(Figure 7.4) (UNEP, 2002)*. Worldwide, approximately

FIGURE 7.4

2002 Urban Dwellers

	Asia	**48%**
	Europe	**19%**
	Latin America/ Caribbean	**14%**
	Africa	**10%**
	North America	**9%**
Source: UNEP, 2002	Total	**2.9 billion**

6% of urban citizens are at risk from inadequate water and 17% from poor sanitation. Africa is most at risk with 14% lacking adequate water and 20% having inadequate sanitation. Asian cities are in a similar position with 7% suffering from poor water and 26%

from poor sanitation. Latin American and Caribbean numbers are slightly better at 6% and 14% for poor water and sanitation. And European and North American populations are — with some minor and intermittent exceptions — relatively secure *(Figure 7.5) (WHO/ UNICEF, 2002)*. Overall, these numbers are likely to understate

FIGURE 7.5

Urban Citizens at Risk in 2002 for Poor Water/Sanitation

	WATER	SANITATION
Africa	14%	20%
Asia	7%	26%
Latin America/ Caribbean	6%	14%
Europe	.4%	1%
North America	0%	0%
Global	6%	17%

Source: WHO/ UNICEF, 2002.

the problem as a result of underreporting, differing definitions of "safe" and "adequate" and considerable variability from nation to nation, city to city and community to community. If one looks at the ideal — piped water and sanitation — it is clear that the challenge, especially in the developing world, is considerable *(Figure 7.6)*.

FIGURE 7.6

2002 Urban Households with Piped Water/Sewers

	PIPED WATER	PIPED SEWERS
Africa	40%	18%
Asia	78%	48%
Latin America/ Caribbean	78%	38%
Oceania	72%	16%
Europe	90%	88%
North America	96%	94%

Source: WHO/ UNICEF, 2002.

HEALTHY WATERS

Sanitation tends to be worse in smaller cities than in large urban settings. A study of 43 cities in Africa showed that only 18% had toilets connected to sewers. In many of the settings, shared toilets or pit latrines were the rule *(Hewett and Montgomery, 2001)*. Shared toilets have a wide range of problems, including cross-contamination, accessibility to flies and other disease-carrying insects, overuse, poor maintenance, travel distance (especially for young children), privacy (especially for women and girls) and expense to utilize public latrines. A study in Ghana in 2000 demonstrated that regular use of public latrines by family members could consume up to 15% of family revenue. Not surprising then that open defecation and paper wrapping of fecal material are not uncommon. A study of children under age 5 in India revealed only 1% use latrines. 5% of parents dispose children's feces into a latrine. The remaining 95% throw them into ditches, streets or yards. In poor settlements, lack of solid waste collection further complicates these practices *(Korboe, 2000)*.

Inadequate drainage and disposal of contaminated waste accumulates and translates into higher direct disease burden and secondary contamination of water sources. Open ditch disposal has to wait only for the next storm to flood surrounding areas with disease, and standing, soggy, polluted materials provide excellent breeding grounds for insect disease vectors.

As cities grow and prosper, water consumption predictably increases. This water is then returned almost always in a lower quality state to lakes, rivers and seas. The water coming from the sanitary systems is joined by wastewater. With backup, the streams of sewage connect and travel. Containment under such circumstance is highly unlikely. Poor segments of the population, from Mamba to Seoul to Delhi, are gradually segregated to smaller districts, usually selected because they are the worst location, least valuable and most compromised. The cost of extending water, sewage and drainage to these areas is prohibitive and low on the priority list considering the fact that many of these settlements are unplanned and unstable.

Urban centers, in concentrating their populations close to coastal waters, are vulnerable as well to water-related disasters, as we saw dramatically with Hurricane Katrina in 2005. Floods cause the major loss of life. Studies reveal that most deaths and injuries could have been prevented with better predictive warnings, preparation and response capability. Drainage infrastructure, good watershed management and well-planned construction and housing offer protection. In contrast, population concentrations in flood paths, flammable shelters and fuel-based cooking and heating ensure higher death and injury tolls.

The water challenges encountered around the world are uniquely different one from another. What they share in common is the need for local governance and site-specific solutions. Good water governance is built around human needs, with institutions tailored to servicing those needs. Good water governance takes a long-term integrated view, supporting industries and developers for economic growth, but setting limits on where and when and how, so that the overall impact on the regional water basin can be managed. Good urban water governance is accountable to the citizens, is properly funded and views basic provision of water and sanitation within these growing urban enterprises as not only equitable and just, but essential to accomplishing the full economic and human potential of the enterprise.

You could not step twice into the same rivers;

for other waters are ever flowing on to you.

— Heraclitus of Ephesus

CHAPTER 8 Natural Water Disasters

No natural disasters in our lifetime generated more powerful and destructive images than did the tsunami that struck Asia and Africa in December 2004 and Hurricane Katrina that hit the U.S. Gulf Coast in August 2005. These two events, in dramatic fashion, illustrated both the power of water and the vulnerability of coastal and river basin populations in the absence of early warning and adequate disaster preparation and response capability.

The story in both cases was not how many died, but rather why they had died and how well would the survivors — well — survive. Early warning systems did not exist or were not heeded, infrastructure was ill-conceived, communication systems were wholly inadequate, safe havens were non-existent and that's just the short list. Long-term impact on quantity and quality of water, how best to prevent secondary epidemics of water-borne diseases, destruction of what infrastructure had existed, homelessness, abandonment of property, environmental losses and economic, social and political impact remain to be tabulated.

These two disasters greatly expanded awareness that water-borne disasters are not inconsequential. Too much water and too little water are not a good thing. Natural disasters in 1999 accounted for over 50,000 deaths worldwide. That loss is not shared equally. 93% of the 1999 loss of life was from the developing world, with only 7% from developed nations. And a single disaster in a developing nation can result in 10% reductions in Gross National Product (GNP) *(UN, 2003)*.

There were 2,200 natural disasters in the last decade of the 20th century. 35% occurred in Asia, 29% in Africa, 20% in the Americas,

13% in Europe and 3% in Oceania. 89% of the natural disasters were water-related, including floods (50%), drought (11%) and water-related epidemics (28%). Only 9% were due to landslides, earthquakes or avalanche, and just 2% from famine. Economic losses from water-related disasters approximate 20% of GNP *(Figure 8.1) (CRED, 2002).*

FIGURE 8.1

**Water-Associated Disasters
1990–2001**

LOCATION	
Asia	35%
Africa	29%
Americas	20%
Europe	13%
Oceania	3%

TYPE	
Flood	50%
Epidemic	28%
Drought	11%
Landslide, Earthquake or Avalanche	9%
Famine	2%

Source: CRED, 2002.

Drivers for disaster include national conflict, weather events, deficient economic, social and political policy and human error. The fact that water planning has been largely non-integrated has amplified the risks and the population vulnerability. The number of natural catastrophes has been steadily growing for a half century, with rises in frequency and intensity of floods, earthquakes, windstorms and volcanic eruptions. Economic losses in 1999 were pegged at $70 billion, up from $30 billion in 1990. Population impacted rose from 147 million to 211 million during the same period *(UN, 2003).*

The majority of the damage has been on the water/weather side, not from geologic events, which have been stable. Water events appear to be tied to changing weather, changed weather to global warming, global warming to CO_2 emissions and to carbonization of our atmosphere. A few facts: In 2004, global emission of carbon exceeded 7 billion metric tons, and is expected to rise to 10.5 billion metric tons by 2029 and 14 billion metric tons by 2054. The United States alone accounted for 20% of the total emissions and 34% of the industrial CO_2 emissions. In fact, the average American in 2004, through his or her actions, generated 12,000 pounds of CO_2. All of this output over the past 100 years of our industrial age has caught up with our atmosphere *(Figure 8.2)*. In 1780, the CO_2 levels in the

FIGURE 8.2

CO_2 Levels in Earth's Atmosphere

	YEAR	PARTS PER MILLION
	1780	280
	1930	315
	1975	330
	1995	360
	2005	380
Source: Kolbert, 2005.	Projected 2050	500

Earth's atmosphere were only 280 parts per million (ppm). Over the next 150 years, levels rose 35 ppm to 315 ppm. But by 1975, we were up to 330 ppm of CO_2, by 1995 had jumped to 360 ppm and by 2005 were at 380 ppm. By 2050, we are expected to double pre-industrialization levels, rising to 500 ppm *(Kolbert, 2005)*. Such levels are difficult if not impossible to reverse, and the negative impact on weather stability at that level is ensured. Asia, as we saw recently, is especially vulnerable. 93% of the flood-caused deaths (228,000) from 1987 to 1996 occurred in Asia. Hurricane Katrina, however, illustrates that developed nations in North America are not immune. Of the people affected by natural disasters, floods accounted for 65% of those affected but only 15% of deaths. Famine, in contrast, accounted for only 20% affected, but was far more deadly, accounting for 42% of deaths between 1973 and 1997 *(UN, 2003)*.

In addition to weather, other risk factors are on the rise. Populations in flood plains are growing in numbers and density. Watershed use is increasingly compromised, lowering our capacity to absorb a portion of the water force impact. Poor people are migrating to vulnerable population centers. Urbanization and deforestation decrease water storage capacity and magnify water volume, speed, soil and waste transport and destructive effect. Dry areas can be especially vulnerable, as preparation is minimal and obstruction to water flow non-existent. Floods also can be useful, when directed away from vulnerable human populations, since they transport nutrients and species as part of important ecological cycles.

If floods are the most visible, dramatic and common water-related disaster, droughts are the most destructive to life. 280,000 deaths from famine in the past decade is a sad number to contemplate. The 1991/1992 drought in sub-Saharan Africa impacted 110 million people over some 7 million square kilometers. Looking back, rather than forward, we had 15 major global droughts in the past 40 years, resulting in 1,761,789 deaths and some 31 trillion (US$) in losses *(Figure 8.3) (Munich Re, 2001)*. Combine drought with conflict, deforestation, overgrazing and human migration, and the human misery index explodes. Trend lines show progressive vulnerability with the current 1 billion living in water-scarce areas expected to rise an additional 140% to 2.4 billion by 2025, affecting 30% of the global population *(IPCC, 2002)*.

The lasting impact of these natural disasters derives from their three-prong attack on economics, environment and social structure. Just looking at the economics can be sobering. The 1990 drought in Zimbabwe, recent floods in Mozambique and the 2000

FIGURE 8.3

Droughts: 1960–2000

YEAR	COUNTRY	FATALITIES	LOSSES (U.S. $ Millions)
1965–1967	India	1,500,000	100
1972–1975	Africa	250,000	500
1976	United Kingdom	—	1,000
1979–1980	Canada	—	3,000
April–June 1988	United States	—	13,000
June–July 1988	China	1,440	—
1989–1990	Angola	10,000	—
Summer 1989	France	—	1,600
January–October 1990	Greece	—	1,300
Summer 1990	Yugoslavia	—	1,000
January–March 1992	Africa	—	1,000
May–August 1998	United States	130	4,275
January–August 1999	Iran	—	3,300
January–April 1999	Mauritius	—	175
June–August 1999	United States	214	1,000

Source: Munich Re, 2001.

drought in Brazil decreased GNP by 11% and 23% in the first two and cut annual projected growth in half in the third. Integrated water resource management mitigates the triple risks and addresses uncertainty in a proactive way *(UN, 2003)*.

Managing risk is about knowing the risk, defining and implementing measures to reduce the risk and spreading the risk through financial systems like insurance. The cost of such instruments decreases as good policies and planning eliminate that portion of the risk under human control. For example, in flood risk reduction there are structural and non-structural adjustments that can decrease risk. Structural change may include construction of dams, channels, flood ways and flood reservoirs, flood dikes, early warning systems, stockpiling of supplies and temporary shelters. A non-structural approach might be land zone planning within natural flood plains. Approaches and contributions are somewhat colored by one's position and point of view. If you are the WHO, there is a focus on emergency-related health hazards. If you are the UN World Food Program (WFP), post-disaster food relief and rehabilitation support is your likely emphasis. If you are the UN Development Program (UNDP), disaster avoidance, prevention and preparedness are your center points. If you are the World Bank, unique financial instruments that mitigate risk and define water resource variability forecasting are special areas of emphasis. And if you are the Global Water Partnership, it's all about Integrated Water Resource Management (IWRM). Similarly, on a local level, each individual and leader has something concrete to contribute. The challenge has been to place them at the same table and keep them there long enough to effect change and get ahead of the curve.

This is not to ignore political realities. Just and Netanyahu in "Conflict and Cooperation on Trans-boundary Water Resources" in 1998 put it this way, "Politicians have the incentive to balance allocations of budgets in a way that preserves political support. Political sustainability is important; and security and stability, together with distributional goals, make up important aspects of political agendas and are often given higher priority than efficiency. Losses to society and the micro-costs imposed on the public could therefore be substantial, but are often disregarded. In the political environment therefore, policy often responds to shorter-term concern than to the long-term consequences to society."

For those in charge, beyond the immediate threat of a water disaster event, there is the issue of restoring water access post-disaster. For those populations dependent on a single source of water or a single route of water delivery, the risks associated with interruption are severe and immediate. Interruption also carries high likelihood of introduction of contaminants into opened systems. Pollution and salination of fresh water bodies can be expected short-term, and ground water contamination from soil-based pollutants is often a long-term issue.

The vulnerable are often poor. Lack of planning means a disaster immediately tips things over the edge. It's a classic case of being in the wrong place at the wrong time. Substandard housing, fragile infrastructure, along a vulnerable flood plain, combined with marginal nutrition and health, make human tragedy a likely outcome. 39% of the disasters that created food emergencies were a function of human-induced rather than natural disasters. This means that at least 4 of 10 food-related emergencies could have been mitigated by better human preparedness and management. Failing to do so costs lives, expands regional tensions and ensures societal instability (UN, 2003).

Increasingly, the impact of inaction is measurable in lives lost, lost GNP, lost growth, lost development, number of lives exposed and affected and percentage of disasters that are human- versus naturally-induced. Such effects help make the case for action rather than inaction and provide predictive trend lines that forecast the extent of the risk and instigate dialogue as to potential causes, such as climactic changes and expanding population growth in vulnerable coastal areas.

Who is responsible makes a big difference. In smaller, more traditional settings, users have historically been hands-on involved in all types of water issues including climactic and economic. But as population and support systems expand, they become more complex and costly, causing responsibility and control to shift to government. Now we are witnessing active exploration of public/private coalitions and a responsibility shift in some locations for day-to-day operations to outsourced services under the control of the private sector. Risk management for natural and man-made disasters often falls between the cracks. Clearly when it comes to threats that are unpredictable and invisible, there is a tendency to defer responsibility and to favor real-time risk-based planning and intervention.

A special challenge exists in trans-boundary areas that are politically unstable. An area such as post-Soviet Central Asia faces stark choices. On one level there is both a risk of natural water disasters that is quite obvious and uncontested, as well as acknowledged standing political tension, even without injecting the complex issue of sustained development. Flipped on its side however, Integrated Water Resource Management, instituting management of the risk of trans-boundary water disasters, provides a challenge that is definable, real and shared. A focused approach in this area not only serves the people but also can build trust equity and the will to take on challenges that are more sensitive and politically explosive.

The long and short of it is that risk of water-related disasters is growing. Absent preparedness, the losses are complex and considerable, measured in human life and the loss of social, economic and environmental capital. Such disasters are increasingly magnified through human error, can occur out of nowhere and generate highly uncoordinated responses. Poor and marginalized populations are most often the victims, with secondary down-cycling of health status a predictable end effect. A decade ago, the emphasis was on the flood and drought itself. Today, the focus is more squarely on the people at risk and affected by these water-related disasters.

We will only know the worth of

water when the well is dry.

— *Benjamin Franklin*

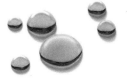

HEALTHY WATERS

CHAPTER 9 # Pricing and Sharing Water

In 1992, The International Conference on Water and the Environment generated the Dublin Statement, highly controversial but also critically relevant if this unique and complex resource is to be both preserved and equitably distributed *(Figure 9.1) (UNEP, 2000)*. The

FIGURE 9.1

The Controversy Over Privatization of Water

	PRO	CON
	· Strengthens information and education.	· Can lead to market dominance.
	· Provides capital.	· May increase prices.
	· Expands data and monitoring.	· Raises significant equity issues.
	· Provides new, efficient technology.	· Has had variable results.
	· Demands a regulatory framework.	· Challenges regulators.
	· Fully values a scarce resource.	· Can lead to profiteering.
Source: UNEP, 2000.		· May be difficult to terminate contracts.

statement reads that: "Water has an economic value in all its competing uses and should be recognized as an economic competing good." It further weighs in on the social implications, leaving no chance for misperception, stating: "It is vital to recognize first the basic right of all human beings to have access to clean water and sanitation at an affordable cost" *(UN, 1992).*

How do people value water? The simple answer is "differently." We know for certain that value is linked to quantity, quality and ability to pay. It is also linked to purpose. Water for drinking, for example, carries a different value than water for laundry washing. How water is priced may also be quite different than the cost of supplying it — or said another way, water may be priced to be affordable to the consumer, with true cost recovered through indirect tariffs or subsidies. For many, water seems to be unlimited and free. As such, incentives for efficiency are relatively non-existent beyond social good and social conscience. This is not to say that societies since the beginning of humankind have not weighed in with rules and approaches to fairly provide enough water at least for survival, and, if plentiful, for other functional purposes as well. They have. But principles that could be generally agreed-upon and utilized as benchmarks within and across geographic boundaries have been largely absent.

At the 1998 Expert Group Meeting for the United Nations Commission for Sustainable Development, certain principles were confirmed. These included: Economics —water planning and management must be integrated into the economy; Allocation — since water is finite and vulnerable, analysis of costs and benefits of different allocations should drive these discussions; Accountability — efficient, transparent responsibility for water management must be assigned, monitored and evaluated; Cost Recovery — all costs must be covered by 2015 to ensure access and sustainability, subsidies may be required and should be transparent; Financing —new financial resources must be marshaled to access water supplies and maximize efficient use of technology to address poverty and the projected new demands for water *(UN, 2003)*.

As we've seen, water serves many different purposes, and is used and reused in various ways, often quite casually and without much thought. Most are conscious of its value in sustaining all life, human and otherwise. Some understand that water plays a vital role in agriculture, industry and energy. Others know it can be drilled for, channeled, diverted, soiled, discarded but not fully lost. Water contributes in many complex ways, each of which carries some economic benefit. Sharing economic information about water can stimulate brisk discussion of both distribution priorities and efficiencies.

The value attributed to water is bound to time and place. It is a local need, and locally provided. For most of us, domestic need for water would trump agricultural need. We highly value a predictable source, and are uncomfortable with tying our lives themselves to good luck or good weather. All life forms are true consumers of water. In contrast, water use for generating hydropower electricity, while not consuming the water itself, does divert it from other uses, thus resulting in its loss for other priorities. As to who is using increasing amounts of water for energy and otherwise, increasingly it is being consumed in urban areas. It is here that populations and industry have formed a symbiotic relationship. Increasingly progress of developing nations is tied to their growing industrial complex. And industry needs water, uses lots of it (now 22% of all withdrawals) and is benefiting from the shift of water away from agriculture (in part due to efficiencies).

There is a cost to poor water management. A study of 15 water and sanitation projects executed in the 1990s with World Bank funds showed that 67% of the projects collapsed in time due to poor management and absent maintenance (UN, 2003). On a much smaller scale, individual "water managers" exerted a similarly large negative economic impact on ground water. When you think about ground water, it's a rather large, invisible, geographically non-definable, incredibly useful resource that multiple individuals can siphon off simultaneously if they own the land above the aquifer. Ground water has been defined as a "common property resource with very high use value." Yet it is limited in one important way. It is an easily damaged resource, vulnerable at many sites, and once damaged does not clean up well. Thus, absent consistent, distributive, enlightened management, the value of this resource long-term is at great risk.

So experts continue to agree that valuing water is complex. Economists develop their formulas, but even the best have trouble putting a price on the intrinsic value of this resource. And while the economist may think she understands it, the language and approach are rarely transferable to real-world situations. For most involved in day-to-day water management, value is all about making wise allocations and establishing more efficient and holistic system management. The supply and demand sides are both behavioral and process engineered. And if the math remains fuzzy, the questions are coming into greater focus. How much efficiency can we deliver and at what economic, social and political cost?

As to the cost, three studies have estimated the total annual global funding requirement to reach the UN Millennium Goals for water and sanitation at between $111 and $180 billion per year *(PriceWaterhouseCoopers, 2001; IUNC, 2002)*. Seeking investment, eyes are increasingly turning to the private sector. The fear of course is that the notion of equitable and just valuing of water will rapidly devolve into discussions of price and profit alone. The more strident warn of bribes, corruption and profiteering. Yet public-private partnerships are growing and citizens are being reassured by their leaders that regulatory checks and balance will prevent abuse. The most critical issues in many eyes are ultimate control of the asset and need for sustained investment.

If the control issue is not fully resolved, there does appear to be a growing consensus regarding the principle of "full cost recovery." This means somebody has to pay for the costs of the water being used. In practical terms, the principle tends to decrease total subsidies, promote cross-subsidization between user groups and place some financial risk (except for those impoverished) on end-users of water. For the largest water consumer — agriculture — accurate pricing stimulates investment in efficient systems and careful monitoring by farmers of service levels of system providers.

These approaches are logical and within reach. Other areas such as tariff restructuring and analyzing the true economic value of a multidistrict river basin are considerably more complex.

On the simplest level, both prices and tariffs recognize the economic value of water. Water is a commodity, affected by supply and demand, by the market, albeit a regulated one. Fair pricing is all over the map. If one compares the water prices for consumers in 5,000 square meters (m^2) of city office space and utilizing at least 10,000 cubic meters (m^3) of water per year, prices vary from a low of .40 US\$/m^3 in Canada to a high of 1.91 US\$/m^3 in Germany *(Figure 9.2)*

FIGURE 9.2

Variations in Water Pricing

	US \$1/m^3	DIFFERENCE FROM CANADA
Canada	.40	—
South Africa	.47	+18%
Australia	.50	+25%
United States	.51	+28%
Spain	.57	+43%
Sweden	.58	+45%
Ireland	.63	+58%
Finland	.69	+73%
Italy	.76	+90%
UK	1.18	+195%
France	1.23	+208%
Netherlands	1.25	+213%
Belgium	1.54	+285%
Denmark	1.64	+310%
Germany	1.91	+378%

Source: Watertech Online, 2001.

(Watertech Online, 2001). Resistance to realistic pricing is in part belief system-driven and in part the absence of scientific, legal and regulatory institutions necessary to accurately apply cost to those who generate waste, inefficiencies and pollution of water.

In many areas, water rights can be traded like real estate. Policy determines the legal options. One community may levy tariffs, another open it up to contractors and the highest bidder. In the developing world, there is a movement toward maximum decentralization to municipal authorities, placing controls and management responsibilities as close to the source and use as possible. If there is a weakness in this approach, it is under-investment and inadequate capacity to execute and maintain a system approach. Capacity includes technical know-how. Choosing the right system can make all the difference in maintenance and sustainability. Well-tested and proven technology is adaptable to different settings, and cost to user can vary multi-fold based on making the right versus the wrong choice in design and equipment. As with all technology, its access and distribution, if not first targeted at those most vulnerable, can actually magnify inequity.

So it is clear that raising the issue of full valuation of such a critical resource is both necessary and controversial. But it is worthwhile to consider the alternative — that is, the status-quo. The UN in its World Water Development Report states, "The legacy of public funded water services in excessive quantities to the few and at subsidized prices has created inefficient conditions resulting in severe environmental impacts on the resource itself. In many regions, the poor already subsidize those richest in society for their water use."

The first step then is to include an economic evaluation in the Integrated Water Management Plan. Such a plan must look at the wide range of opportunity costs and the impact, both positive and negative, of pursuing a list of priorities. The introduction of market-based and participating approaches requires policy changes and, at times, new management and governance. Integration is the crux since we are dealing with a fixed resource and expanding demand. Maximizing the benefit to individuals, families, communities and societies is the challenge. But, remember, water flows. So to make this all work, to truly create Integrated Water Resource

Management, implies a level of stable and long-term human cooperation that, till now, has escaped our reach.

We must therefore learn to share — share between individuals, share between sectors, share between jurisdictions. To share implies a holistic view. It implies advance planning and preparedness. It implies recognizing the value of an essential and limited resource. Sharing may seem a minor issue if you are upstream, but it is clearly of unparalleled importance if you are downstream. Water may be shared directly or as "virtual water" in a trade for agricultural or manufactured products.

There are examples currently of planned sharing of water, almost by necessity. Take China, exploding economically and socially over the past two decades. Early on, the government appreciated that water, if managed poorly, could be their Achilles' heel. Looking at their water resources, they saw a per capita supply of water that was only 25% of the global average. The numbers were the numbers: annual average precipitation, 648 millimeters (mm); annual runoff, 2,712 cubic kilometers (km³), ground water reserves, 829 km³, total water resources, 2,812 km³. A huge population supported by only the sixth largest accessible water supply, and to make things worse a supply plagued by uneven distribution. And on the demand side: population growing, agriculture growing and industry on fire. First step, make agriculture use water efficiently. The result, with only 7% of its land planted, China reliably feeds its people, who represent 22 percent of the global population. With agricultural water use flat, total water volume use in 2000 reached 550 km³, with approximately 10% for domestic use, 67% for agriculture and 21% for industrial use. Just as manufacturing has grown, so has demand increased and competition with farmers and others is on the rise. The response has been the creation of the Water Conservation Scheme, creating standards for water conservation, management practices, flood control, disaster preparedness and ongoing allocation priorities proactively *(UN, 2003)*. The learning? Sharing is hard work.

And sharing can be expensive. Short-term thinkers spent a couple of decades drawing water off the Florida Everglades. There are a lot of good reasons not to mess with your wetlands, like having a place for floodwater to collect and maintaining species diversity. But add to this that tourism in Florida is a $20 billion business, and visitors weren't enthusiastic about a dried-up Everglades. So Florida has decided to reverse the damage, reclaiming and restoring some 1 million hectares (a hectare is the customary metric unit of land equal to 100 acres) of ecosystem, and in the process generating an additional 700 cubic millimeters (mm^3) of fresh water a day. Florida is learning to share with itself — and its challenge is easy compared with the Danube River watershed, running through 18 countries on its way to the Black Sea *(UN, 2003)*. The Danube Regional Project must be endorsed and empowered by enabling legislation and proactive policies in all countries. Sharing here is complex but possible. In fact, when it comes to water, nations have generally been cooperative. Many have national agreements on intersectional allocation, financial incentives through tariffs and subsidies, management of abstraction rates and volumes, sites, reservoir rules and quality objectives.

Most water managers look at the watershed as the unit of management quite independent of geographic boundaries. Over the years, bridges with neighbors were most easily built first by sharing information and by encouraging an open platform that invited everyone's participation. Management structures, rules for allocation and commitment to values like equity then followed. Still, water and all its ramifications certainly challenge intergovernmental political capacity.

There are 263 trans-boundary water basins involving 145 different nations *(International Riverbasin Registry, 2002)*. One third of these basins are shared between two or more countries, and 19 of the basins unite five or more countries. The Danube River has 18. Potential disputes over water between countries in the past 50 years have numbered 1,831 around the globe, 27% marked by anger and acrimony and 73% marked by cooperation and focus on the solution according to a 2001 study by Oregon State University *(UN, 2003)*. Of the 1,831 around the globe, only 2% involved violence. Over the past 50 years, 200 successful water agreements were endorsed, and since AD 805, there have been 3,600 water treaties tied to international water agreements. So the record is clear. When it comes to water, nations, even those in conflict with each other, have found a way to get along. One dramatic example is the Mekong Committee which was established in 1957 and remained functional throughout the entire Vietnam War *(UN, 2003)*.

When trouble does arise, it generally is from lack of a trans-boundary structure or from unilateral action by one party without informing a second affected party. Sharing is about institutional capacity-building and preventive diplomacy. In the last 10 years, there have been 16 new multinational water treaties signed. The treaties have increased in quantity and quality. Most now include specifics about shared allocations, water-quality monitoring, basin-wide participation and, in some cases, formal water commissions with governance powers.

Surface water management continues to outpace ground water management due to the latter's hidden nature and lack of a legal framework. Aquifers worldwide provide access to drinking water to 1.5 billion people. The major threats are overpumping and pollution *(Figure 9.3)* *(UNEP, 2000)*. Consider for example that there are over 100 trans-boundary aquifers in Europe alone. Focus

FIGURE 9.3

Ground Water Aquifers Highlights

Use:	
	· Aquifers provide access for drinking water and domestic use to 1.5 billion people.
Threats:	
	· Overpumping:
	—Withdrawal of water can be greater than recharge.
	· Pollution:
	—Caused by poor sanitation, industrial discharge and agricultural runoff.
	· Damage:
	—Aquifers are costly or impossible to repair.

Source: P, 2000.

on ground water will surely expand as the science and imaging of their stores become more ubiquitous, and as their connection to river basins, wetlands and other elements of the hydrological cycle become better understood. The issues will be at least as complex as those for surface water. Discharge into a single aquifer may occur commonly on one side of the border, while recharge is on the other. Support for wetlands and biodiversity also must be considered, along with sustainable support for domestic, agricultural, industrial and energy needs. As the database grows, the issue of ground water will come into greater focus, and what is hidden and subconscious now will rise up and demand conscious and wise oversight.

Drawing on recent history, however, we have reason to be optimistic that preventive hydro-diplomacy will rise. Lessons already learned include that management structures must be adaptable and flexible; criteria for allocations need to be transparent and non-rigid; public input must be pursued and considered; social equity cannot be ignored. In regard to this last learning, the monitoring of water availability per person, percentage of water originating beyond state borders, supply/demand consumption rates and strategic reliance on hydroelectric for energy help predict the potential for conflict.

As interdependency continues to grow, the record shows that managing and governing water, more often than not, can be a source of expansion of social, cultural and political capital between nations rather than withdrawal of these resources. The investment then pays off in the short and long term on many levels. It forces nations to come to grips with their values and priorities using valuation of water as a proxy, and challenges their leaders to design durable political and legal structures that codify the capacity to share in a common future.

Such nations, at the least, currently share our oceans. International governance of our oceans is slowly progressing, as are some 145 different nations that are criss-crossed by 268 trans-boundary water basins. In addition, many national, regional and local bodies have struggled to provide a structure to fairly govern the issue of water. What are they all seeking? First, comprehensive policies that are holistic, integrated and environmentally sound. Second, strong institutions able to improve water laws. And third, an integrated approach that is "dynamic, interactive and multisectoral" and one capable of embracing all water users in a socioeconomic plan.

By now most recognize that rules and regulations mean little absent enforcement. What are territories addressing right now? Incoherency, fragmentation, inadequacy and misplaced incentives related to water property rights. Good governance promises and must deliver an integrated participatory approach. Some structures focus on financial accountability and management. Others on efficiency alone. But, on a larger level, this is about participatory democracy to ensure fundamental provision of human rights.

The United Nations Development Program (UNDP) defines governance as "the exercise of economic, political and administrative authority to manage a country's affairs at all levels. It comprises the mechanisms, processes and institutions through which citizens and groups articulate their interests, exercise their legal rights, meet their obligations and mediate their differences" *(UNDP, 1997)*.

When the concept of governance is applied to water, roles, issues and equitable policy immediately surface for discussion *(Figure 9.4)*. The

FIGURE 9.4

Water Governance Discussion Points

Equity:	• There is a need for holistic and integrated approaches that fairly balance use.
Roles:	• There is a need for clarification of stakeholders, economic incentives, standards and conflict resolution.
Issues:	• There is a need to consider pricing, incentives, levels of regulation and bureaucratic structure.

Source: UN, 2003.

establishment of water institutions create the capacity to define who gets what, when they get it and how they get it. It also defines and balances economic and social gain. There are certain basic tenets that must now be embraced, including participation, transparency, clarity, accountability, responsibility, integration, equity and justice *(UN, 2003)*.

Critical to initiation of sustainable water governance is addressing up-front who owns the water. "Own" here is not a clear concept. Water rights are most often tied to property law. But the resource is variable, is often shared and generates a multiplicity of claims. Illegal abstraction is not uncommon and can be difficult to identify, let alone adjudicate. The solution is to establish the context of water as a common resource system and acknowledge that water is an increasingly scarce resource. When water is treated solely as a property right, those with property are empowered to exclude those without property from access to water. Private ownership of the land provides private control of the surface water above and the ground water below. Without regulation or guidance, those with property or finances are advantaged to the extreme. This is not to say that public control of the resource ensures more equitable distribution. In fact, history indicates otherwise. If one is poor, isolated or immobilized, and especially if the public systems are poorly conceived, underfunded and not maintained, the results can and have been disastrous.

Governance is part of the picture, backed up by good policy and enlightened legislation. Such governance reflects a tripartite vision of sustainability, efficiency and equity. But increasingly, to deliver the goods requires good management in the form of assessment, measurement, data analysis and decision management systems, as well as technology support. When these capabilities are accessed by a public-private partnership and function on the local catchbasin level, allocations, efficiency and environmental sustainability can be addressed. Handled wisely, the water governance pyramid can deliver social equity *(Figure 9.5)*. According to the Global Water Partnership, as noted in the UN Development Report, Integrated Water Resource

FIGURE 9.5

Water Governance Pyramid

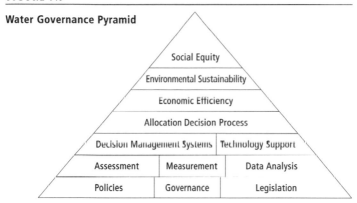

Management (IWRM) "promotes participatory approaches, demand and catchment area management, partnerships, subsidiarity and decentralization, the need to strike a gender balance, the environmental, economic and social value of water and basin or catchment management. It replaces the traditional, fragmented sectorial approach to water management that has led to poor services and unsustainable resource use" *(Figure 9.6) (UN, 2003; GWP, 2000a).*

FIGURE 9.6

Principles of IWRM

1. Organized at catchment level.
2. Integrates water and environment.
3. Focuses on systems and processes.
4. Maximizes stakeholder participation, especially women.
5. Based on knowledge and information.
6. Utilizes best technology and practices.
7. Supports equitable allocation.
8. Considers social, economic and political dimensions.
9. Fully values water as a resource.
10. Builds capacity with sustained financing.

Source: GWP, 2000a.

That is a long way of saying that water is connected to every-thing and everyone. If we can figure out how to manage it well, we will have figured out how to manage ourselves well. The government approach as dictator has not worked. So increasingly government is assuming the responsibility to activate, facilitate and provide focus. On what? On assessment, communication, allocation, conflict resolution, controls, economic instruments and technology — in the hope of overcoming traditional obstacles to integrated manage-ment *(Figure 9.7) (UNEP, 2002)*. Government is also driving home

FIGURE 9.7

Obstacles to IWRM

	1. Weak funding.
	2. Segmented responsibilities:
	· Surface water, ground water, wastewater.
	· Urban water management, urban planning, industrial development.
	3. Disconnect between land use and water use.
	4. Non-optimization of workplace.
	5. Weak education, training and awareness.
Source: UNEP, 2002.	6. Perfect is the enemy of good.

the need to plan water, sanitation and hygiene as one. Changing the institutions requires changing attitudes and behaviors. After all, "one man's waste is another man's job."

As for the private side, the UN Ministerial Declaration at Bonn in 2001 encouraged private sector participation, not as owner, but with a larger roll in financing, managing, operating and maintain-ing water and wastewater systems. This can take on varying forms. In England and Wales, the government maintains regulatory control of water through the Office of Water Services (which has limited prices), The Environmental Agency (focused on allocation and waste/pollution discharge) and the Drinking Water Inspectorate (quality control). With this structure in place protecting the public's interests, private sector industry owns the water infrastructure and plants, and provides financing, operations and maintenance. Other approaches include limited time concessions to private vendors for management, operation and development with governments maintaining ownership as in France (UN, 2003).

In the developing world, private investment and involvement in water management has delivered success but also controversy. Criticisms include secrecy, downgrades on initial service contracts, discontinuation of service and tariff increases. Greatest success has occurred in the more affluent urban areas where capacity to serve and capacity to pay are high. But for urban and rural poor, success requires cross subsidy to allow acceptable private return on investment. In this area, non-governmental organizations (NGOs) have become more visible delivery partners, but they too have been criticized for inconsistent service delivery. In truth, then, there remains no single blueprint. We do know, however, that poor financing and inconsistent, fragmented leadership are most certainly predictors of failure. Complexity is the issue and how best to manage it on the local level. Contributing issues have been outlined in preceding chapters: multiuse, urbanization, poor land management, agricultural pesticides and runoff, deforestation, animal feed lots, failed sanitation policy, wastewater diversion, mining and more. Absent management, the impact is clear and includes declining water quality and quantity, increased water treatment cost, increased water-borne diseases, decreased ground water reserves and ecosystem health, increased siltation and salination of fresh water supplies and degradation of basin and coastal lands.

There is a renewed focus on identifying areas of opportunity (Figure 9.8) (UN, 2003). These include sites where readiness, simplicity, flexibility and community can intersect. Whether a waste minimization club, low water use sanitation scheme or activation of water use association, participation on the local level is a common denominator. It's been said that "Water in a reservoir or an

FIGURE 9.8

Opportunities for IWRM

	1. Simple, realistic, evolutionary projects.
	2. Adaptive management:
	• Flexible, step-wise approach.
	3. Virtual centers of excellence.
	4. Incentivize resource conservation.
	5. "Cradle to grave" lifecycle analysis.
	6. Waste minimization clubs.
	7. Integrated urban water management.
	8. "South to south" partnerships.
	9. Dry/low water use sanitation.
Source: UN, 2003.	10. Involve professional water associations.

aquifer is, in a way, equivalent to money in the bank." If this is true, it only makes good sense to ensure the governance and ongoing investment to prevent untimely withdrawals or catastrophic break-downs that would effectively empty our water bank accounts.

Freedom alone is not enough

without light to read at night,

without time or access to water

to irrigate your farm,

without the ability to catch fish

to feed your family.

— Nelson Mandela

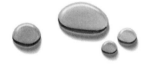

HEALTHY WATERS

Reflecting once again, at the end of this process, on my United Nations friend's question, "What do you really know about water?," I can honestly reply, "More than I knew before."

I knew of course that water was essential to all life. But I was not conscious of the level of interconnectedness and interdependence of our water resources. I was surprised to learn that less than 1% of our water stores are both fresh and accessible, and how critical a challenge we face in keeping our surface and ground waters safe and pure. I was embarrassed to learn that a Masai tribesman survives on an average of less than 5 liters of water a day, while a Los Angelean routinely consumes 100 times this amount. I was surprised as well to realize that where the water sources are does not necessarily match up with population concentrations.

Before work on this project, I had little understanding of the concept of "virtual water," nor the relative amounts of water required to produce quantities of vegetables, grains and meat. That the average global citizen's daily diet represents the consumption of 3,000 liters of water was an eye opener. I knew, of course, that farms consume water, but did not understand that 70% of our supplies are so dedicated, and did not appreciate how successful and critical high-tech irrigation has become. With irrigated fields producing 400% greater food yields than rain-fed fields, with high-tech seeds and advanced agricultural planning, it is no wonder that the world's food supply, except for pockets around the globe, is now relatively secure. And by 2030, 70% of our grain crops are projected to come from irrigated lands; more cause to closely follow land-use issues, pesticide runoff and overall agricultural consumption of water.

The information on aquaculture was fascinating, that today 27% of all the fish we eat is "grown" and that consumption of fish continues to increase rapidly. What is less visible is the potential impact on marine and inland waters from the outputs of "fish farms," and the large amount of marine fish stores that must be caught to feed the fish we "grow." Three pounds of fish food to grow one pound of farmed salmon certainly attracted my attention; as did the power of consumers to drive the agricultural and aquacultural "crop" selections through informed choices of what they eat. When it comes to "growing," countries like China are clearly on the rise, managing to feed their enormous population and weave together a multi-tasked approach like growing rice and fish in the same fields. But at the same time, water availability clearly does not match up with population growth. So China is already in a water-scarcity environment. Over the next 20 years many of us will join their citizens, with an estimated 3.4 billion of our global population projected to be water scarce by 2025.

At the end of this work, I am much more aware of the health linkages between water, sanitation and hygiene. It's amazing that one-sixth of us lack improved water and two-fifths of us lack improved sanitation. And it is understandable that if it's a choice between good water and good sanitation, water wins out, at least in the short term. Clearly our future potential is tied to geography and to gender. It was fascinating to learn that we are just beginning to listen more carefully to women's advice on water policy. The burden that they have carried in the water arena has been heavy indeed. Not surprisingly, when it comes to water, women get it. They understand that without sanitary systems, the water they do have is compromised. They understand that water proximity impacts their productivity. They understand that sanitation facilities at schools that do not secure privacy, especially for girls, ensure lost primary education and lost opportunity. They under-stand that schools provide a dual service in educating and promot-ing health. And they understand that poor water and disease have made an unholy alliance through history, taking target at women and the young and the vulnerable. To accept that 25% of all deaths worldwide and 50% of all hospitalized patients are the result of water-borne diseases is a painful admission.

Through this work, I have gained a better understanding of where we are going as a global family. Clearly we are heading to the cities, and our fate remains to be determined. What we do know is that by 2025, 60% of us will live in cities. Many of these cities still exist on coastal waterways and along major river catchbasins. The number and size of these cities are growing. With proper investment, rural people flooding in may benefit from more secure water and sanita-tion. But without sustained investment and wise policy, they may encounter squalor, disease and water-borne disasters rather than hope and progress.

As we centralize, urbanize and industrialize, I now can see that energy will be a critical lever. And it seems that hydroenergy, well planned, executed and maintained, could help break the cycle of carbonization of our atmosphere and give us some breathing room from global warming. But this would require a much more aggressive cross-sector commitment to clean, non-fossil fuels. I was impressed that almost 20% of the world's energy now comes from hydropower and that by 2010 small hydropower development is expected to grow by a further 60%.

I have now, at the end of this project, a different vision of our planet. Earth, covered in vast oceans of water, is actually a quite fragile planet, requiring care and wise policy. The watershed catchbasins that cover 45% of our land and sustain 60% of our global popula-tion are surprisingly complex and vulnerable. I suspected that these waterways in developing nations would be at risk, but was surprised to learn that 70% of industrial waste and 90% of raw sewage is discharged untreated into the developing world's surface waterways. And in developed nations, zoning and planning vagaries that allow sanitary systems and ground water to cross paths; lack of attention to runoff, deforestation and hog plant manure gone wild; and lackadaisical attention to water quality monitoring, safe food preparation, proper hand washing in hospitals; and the disastrous failure of the response to Hurricane Katrina in the United States all suggest that when it comes to water and health, we all have plenty of room for improvement.

I now have a clearer picture in my mind of surface water and ground water. Most impressive are the many river catchbasins that 145 nations now share, and that the fate of those downstream is largely determined by the behavior of those upstream. Equally intriguing are the vast stores of ground water which will likely be more accurately imaged, managed and efficiently accessed in the future thanks to advanced technology. Once again, these aquifers are shared, sometimes unknowingly, across geographic borders and from the surface appear safe from spoilage or rapid evaporation. But once fouled by pollutants, as I have learned, they may be out of commission for a lifetime, since clean-up can be impossible. And I was surprised to learn that some aquifers in fossil rock are never rechargeable. I didn't know that.

The tsunami of 2004 had already alerted me to the magnitude and power of water disasters. But I was surprised to learn that more than a half a million people had died from water-related disasters in the last decade of the 20th century. This work helped me better understand how man-made and natural disasters are tied to water, climate, pollution and poor preparedness. I also have learned that people will respond to need, especially if the need is caused by an act of nature, is publicized and is urgent and unexpected. But we are less likely to be there if the disaster is the result of human ignorance or malice. It was reassuring to see that throughout history water has generally brought people and nations together. We have made treaties and made peace most of the time. Humans seem better able to cooperate around water than most anything else, suggesting that our world, so in need of common vision and purpose, so fearful and in turmoil, might ride the wave of healthy waters to a better and more secure place.

Finally, I have learned what IWRM means. When I first read the term, Integrated Water Resource Management, my mind wanted to dissect it. Integrated, I learned, has multiple meanings. Water is remarkably connected to everything else — to our environment and ecology, to agriculture and famine, to industry and urbanization, to energy production of all sorts, to weather and weather events and to the health and advancement of all life, including ourselves. Integrated also reflects a system of competing demands and needs that must be harmonized and prioritized if our fixed supply of water is to be able to keep pace with the growing demands of an expanding human population. After all, in the past 100 years our population has tripled, and our water consumption has increased six-fold.

IWRM also positions water as the resource it truly is: valuable, critical, essential to life. If we fail to assign this resource a value, we encourage waste and destruction of this scarce asset. On the other hand, if it is viewed simply as a commodity, we risk further victimizing our most vulnerable brothers and sisters. I have learned that a one dollar investment in water as a resource has an economic return of up to 34 times. But I now understand that the accessible delivery of clean, pure water and the safe discharge of waste require investment of time, energy and money, in a sustained manner. So the challenge is to bridge the gap between a foolish level of waste and incompetence on the one hand, and an unenlightened and inequitable commodity-driven system on the other.

To address this challenge, IWRM preaches management, not just the ordinary type, but a form of management that challenges governments, industry, academics and non-governmental organizations to lend their best talent on behalf of water. In short, we must work together. Beyond a common understanding of the strengths and capabilities of each sector, and the desire for collaboration reflected in a willingness to mutually plan, to align goals and objectives and to share risk, there remains the issue of readiness for IWRM. What are the factors that must be in place to ensure success?

First, if it is true that all politics are local, so too are all successful cross-sector partnerships in so far as they acknowledge in their planning, design and management the realities of time, place, people, culture and institutions in the target geography.

Second, in any cross-sector initiative in health, there should be some level of representation from each of the four sectors: government, non-government, industry and academia. Water is certainly a well-defined common need and public purpose that unites us.

Third, the proposed project or solution must be right-sized to the problem or challenge at hand. Too small and the effort will lack resources to ensure measurability and sustainability. Too large and the effort will create structure without solution.

Fourth, human conditions must be right. This includes identifiable optimistic leaders with the time and willingness to commit and a reservoir of good will among the players to support both innovation and implementation of the common vision, the structural integration, the joint governance and ongoing civic engagement.

Fifth, there needs to be accurate information and baseline data that clearly define the challenges and serve as a grounding for future reasonable outcomes. It is not enough to marshal human resources. There must be an established organizational capacity, processes and oversight to ensure that the human effort translates into a highly coordinated and effective service result. All of which is to say that success in IWRM involves harmonization of diverse needs and interests.

What I have learned is that IWRM has social, political and economic dimensions that directly impact human health, poverty levels and gender equality. IWRM requires reliable data and careful valuation of water as a resource. Identifying the true cost of safe water and sanitation is essential for financing and creating sustainable and reliable infrastructure.

I have learned a lot, certainly more than I knew before. But I continue to be somewhat plagued by my initial admission to the question "How much do you really know about water?" After 30 years in medicine, shouldn't I have known more? Perhaps. But for physicians, nurses and other health professionals in developed nations (excluding those directly involved in public health careers), water has been largely an environmental rather than a health issue — and someone else's responsibility.

Yet today, health for an individual is about having the opportunity to reach one's full human potential, and for a nation, it is the leading edge of development. Health is about wellness and prevention, growth and stability, peace and security. It is about individuals, families, communities and societies looking after each other, caring for and about each other and securing each other's future. What I have learned in this process is that we, as caregivers, need to ride water's wave, because its destination is health, and patients worldwide have the right to expect our active involvement and participation in this critical health issue.

So, where might we begin? *Figure 10.1* and *Figure 10.2* list some possible starting points for health professionals and health partners in both developed and developing nations. But as we move forward, it is increasingly clear that, as all water is interconnected, so too are we as humans. Our fates are linked. We, as caregivers, must move toward the issue in order to secure safety, opportunity, fairness and a better place for all.

FIGURE 10.1

Water Activities for Health Professionals in Developing Nations

1. Seek representation on national and regional IWRM committees.

2. If an IWRM committee does not exist, advocate for its creation.

3. Challenge multinational and home-grown industry to demonstrate water and sanitation leadership.

4. Create and distribute an annual water health report.

5. Advocate for inclusion of women in IWRM committees.

6. Advocate for high-impact, low-cost, point-of-use filtration for drinking water.

7. Examine sanitation facilities at schools to ensure they are adequate and protect privacy.

8. Advocate for universal access and participation in primary education, and ensure the presence of an aggressive health and hygiene curriculum.

9. Monitor average travel distance for water by citizens, and design and implement programs to improve access time.

10. Advocate for and monitor success of water disease surveillance and water disaster preparedness.

FIGURE 10.2

Water Activities for Health Professionals in Developed Nations

1. Understand local zoning laws for wells and sanitation systems, as well as systems for monitoring and enforcement.

2. Promote water policy inclusion in professional school curriculum, promote hospital hand washing.

3. Support research analysis into harmful algal blooms, organohalogens, heavy metals and inorganic compounds, and their impact on coastal waters.

4. Advocate annual well water testing, and food and restaurant health monitoring and surveillance.

5. Create pocket guides to promote choice of ocean-friendly seafood and water-efficient nutrients.

6. Host a water scientist presentation at a health association meeting, focusing on the state of the region's water.

7. Discuss water and health with local industry, encouraging and soliciting their leadership ideas.

8. Understand the status of the region's water disaster preparedness plans.

9. Support efforts to decrease CO_2, mercury and lead emissions.

10. Examine water, sanitation and hygiene standards of public and private schools.

When you drink the water, remember the spring.

— *Chinese proverb*

REFERENCES

Abramovitz, J. 2001. *Unnatural Disasters*. Washington DC, Worldwatch Paper 158, Worldwatch Institute.

Ball, P. 1999. *H_2O: The Biography of Water*. Condon. Phoenix/Orion.

Barraqué, B. *What Can the United Nations Do to Preserve and Promote Freshwater Resources?* http://www.un.org/Pubs/chronicle/2003/issue1/0103p46.html.

Bartone, C.; Bernstein, J.; Leitmann, J.; Eigen, J. 1994. *Towards Environmental Strategies for Cities: Policy Considerations for Urban Environmental Management in Developing Countries*. UNDP/UNCHS/World Bank Urban Management Program, No. 18. Washington DC, World Bank.

Broad, WJ. 1997. *The Universe Below: Discovering the Secrets of the Deep Sea*. New York, Simon and Schuster.

Bryson, Bill. *A Short History of Nearly Everything*. New York, Broadway Books. 2003.

Cosgrove, W.J. and Rijsberman, F.R. 2000. *World Water Vision: Making Water Everybody's Business*. London, World Water Council, Earthscan Publications Ltd.

Costanza, R.; d'Arge, R.; de Groot, R.; Farber, S.; Grasso, M.; Hannon, B.; Limburg, K.; Naeem, S.; O'Neill, R.; Paruelo, J.; Raskin, R.; Sutton, P.; van den Belt, M. 1997. 'The Value of the World's Ecosystem Services and Natural Capital', *Nature*. Vol. 387, pp. 253–60.

CRED (Centre for Research on the Epidemiology of Disasters). 2002. *The OFDA/CRED International Disaster Database*. Brussels, Université Catholique De Louvain.

CSE (Center for Science and the Environment). 1999. *The Citizens Fifth Report*.

Danis, M. 1995. *Institutional Framework for Electricity Supply to Rural Communities: A Literature Review*. University of Cape Town, Energy and Development Research Centre.

Dennis, J. 1996. *The Bird in the Waterfall. A Natural History of Oceans, Rivers and Lakes*. New York, Harper Collins.

Doog, JC. On the Study of Water. *Hydrological Sciences Journal*. Vol 28. (Quoted in UN, 2003.)

Dublin Statement. 1992. Official Outcome of the International Conference on Water and the Environment: Development Issues for the 21st Century, 26–31 January 1992, Dublin. Geneva, World Meteorological Organization.

Economist. 1998. "*The Sea*." May 23, 1998.

ECOSOC (United Nations Economic and Social Council) and CSD (Com-mission on Sustainable Development). 2001. *Water: A Key Resource for Sustainable Development. Report of the Secretary General.* New York, United Nations.

EEC (European Economic Community). 2000. *Framework Directive in the Field of Water Policy (Water Framework). Directive 2000/60/EC of the European Parliament and of the Council of 23 October 2000, Establishing a Framework for EEC Action in the Field of Water Policy.* [Official Journal L327, 22.12.200.] (Quoted in UN, 2003.)

EPA. 2005. *Nonpoint Source Pollution: The Nation's Largest Water Quality Problem.* http://www.epa.gov/owow/nps/facts/point1.htm.

FAO (Food and Agricultural Organization). Aquastat. 2002. http://www.fao.org/ag/agl/aglw/aquastat/main/index.stm.

———. 2002. *World Agriculture: Towards 2015/2030, an FAO Study.* Rome.

———. 2001a. *Crops and Drops. Making the Best Use of Water for Agriculture.* Rome.

———. 2001b. *The State of Food Insecurity in the World.* Rome.

———. 2000. *The State of the World Fisheries and Aquaculture.* Rome.

———. 1997a. *Water Resources of the Near East Region. A Review.* Rome.

———. 1997b. 'Irrigation Potential in Africa. A Basin Approach', *FAO Land and Water Bulletin.* Vol. 4. Rome.

Federal Ministry for the Environment, Nature Conservation and Nuclear Safety, and Federal Ministry for Economic Co-operation and Development. 2001. *Ministerial Declaration, Bonn Keys, and Bonn Recommendation for Action.* Official outcomes of the International Conference on Freshwater, 3–7 December 2001, Bonn.

Gordon, A.L. 2005. *The Climate System: Ocean Stratification.* Columbia University Earth's Environmental Systems. http://eesc.ldeo.columbia.edu/courses/ees/climate/lectures/o_strat.html.

Gleick, P.H. 1993. *Water in Crisis: A Guide to the World's Fresh Water Resources.* New York, Oxford University Press.

GWP (Global Water Partnership). 2000a. *Toward Water Security: A Framework for Action to Achieve the Vision for Water in the 21st Century.* Stockholm.

———. 2000b. *Integrated Water Resources Management.* Technical Advisory Committee Background Paper No. 4 (GWP-TAC4). Stockholm.

Health Politics. 2004. *Healthy Waters: A Public Trust.* www.healthpolitics.com/archives.asp?previous=healthy_water.

———. 2005. *The Lessons We Can Learn from the Tsunami.* http://www.healthpolitics.com/archives.asp?previous=learn_tsunami.

Hidalgo L. *Aral Sea poison dust danger.* BBC News. February 18, 2000.

Hewett, PC and Montgomery, M. 2001. *Poverty and Public Services in Developing Country Cities.* Policy Research Division Working Paper No. 154. New York. Population Council.

Hoeg, K. 2000. DAMS: *Essential Infrastructure for Future Water Management*. Paper presented at the Second World Water Forum for the International Commission on Large Dams. 17-22 March 2000, The Hague.

ICOLD (International Commission on Large Dams). 1994. *Dams and the Environment: Water Quality and Climate*. Paris.

IFRC (International Federation of Red Cross and Red Crescent Societies). 2001. *World Disasters Report 2001*. Geneva.

IHA (International Hydropower Association). Small scale hydrosection. http://europa.eu.int/comm/dgs/energy_transport/index_en.html. May 2002.

Institute of Medicine. 2004. *From Source Water to Drinking Water*. Workshop Summary.

International Journal on Hydropower and Dams. 1997. *1997 Atlas of Hydropower and Dams*. United Kingdom. Awua Media International Ltd. (Quoted in UN, 2003.)

International Riverbasin Registry. 2002. In *United Nations World Water Development Report 2003*. p.304-311.

IPCC (International Programme on Climate Change). 2002. *Climate Change 2001: Synthesis Report*. Geneva. International Programme on Climate Change Secretariat. World Meteorological Organization.

IUCN (International Union for the Conservation of Nature and Natural Resources). 2000. *Vision for Water and Nature. A World Strategy for Conservation and Sustainable Management of Water Resources in the 21st Century — Compilation of All Project Documents*. Cambridge.

IUNC (The World Conservation Union). 2002. *Johannesburg Programme of Action*. A Document prepared for the World Summit on Sustainable Development. (WSSD). 28 August–4 September. Johannesburg.

Just, RE and Netanyahu, S. 1998. *Conflict and Cooperation on Transboundary Water Resources*. Boston, Kluwer Academic Publishers.

Kalbermatten, J.-M.; Julius, D.-S.; Gunnerson, C.-G. 1980. *Appropriate Technology for Water Supply and Sanitation: A Review of the Technical and Economic Options*. Washington DC, The World Bank.

Kenchington, RA. 2003. *Managing Marine Environments: An Introduction to Issues of Sustainability, Conservation, Planning and Implementation*. In: Conserving Marine Environments: Out of Site, Out of Mind. Pat Hutchings and Dan Lunney (eds.). Royal Zoological Society of New South Wales. Mosman, NSW Australia.

Kolbert, E. 2005. *The Climate of Man–III: What Can Be Done?* The New Yorker, May 9, 2005.

Korboe, D., et al. 2000. *Urban Governance, Partnership and Poverty: Kumasi*. In Urban Governance Partnership and Poverty Working Paper 10. Birmingham, International Development Department, University of Birmingham. (Quoted in UN, 2003.)

Korzun, V., et al. *Atlas of the World Water Balance*. USSR National Committee for the IHD (International Hydrological Decade) Gidromet: English translation.

1974. Paris, UN Educational, Scientific and Cultural Organization. (Quoted in UN, 2003.)

Margulis, L and Sagan, D. 1986. *Microcosmos. Four Billion Years of Evolution from Our Microbial Ancestors.* New York, Summit Books.

Mazoyer, M. and Roudart, L. 1998. *Histoire des Agricultures du Monde, du Neolithique a la Crise Contemporine.* Paris, Editions du Seuil. (Quoted in UN, 2003.)

McCarthy, J.J.; Canziani, O.F.; Leary, N.A.; Dokken, D.J.; White, K.S. 2001. *Climate Change 2001. Impacts, Adaptation, and Vulnerability.* Cambridge, Cambridge University Press.

Meybeck, M. 1979. *Concentration des Eaux Fuviales en Elements Majeurs et Appoits en Solution aux Oceans.* Revue de Geologie Dynamique et de Geographie Physique. Vol. 21, pp.215-46. (Quoted in UN, 2003.)

Ministerial Declaration of The Hague on Water Security in the 21st Century. 2001. Official Outcome of the Second World Water Forum, 3–7 December 2001, The Hague.

Montgomery, M. 2002. *Analysis of 86 Demographic and Health Surveys Held in 53 Different Nations Between 1986 and 1998.* New York, Population Council. (Quoted in UN, 2003.)

Munich Re. 2001. *Topics, Annual Review: Natural Catastrophes 2000.* Munich.

New Yorker. CO₂ Article. 2005.

Postel, S. 1993. 'Water and Agriculture'. In: P.H. Gleick (ed.), *Water in Crisis: A Guide to the World's Fresh Water Resources.* New York, Oxford University Press.

Postel, S. L.; Daily, G. C.; Ehrlich, P. R. 1996. "Human Appropriation of Renewable Fresh Water." *Science,* Vol. 271, pp. 785–8.

PricewaterhouseCoopers. 2001. *Water: a World Financial Issue — A Major Challenge for Sustainable Development in the 21st Century.* Sustainable Development Series. Paris.

Reuter, L.; Falk, H.; Groat, C.; Coussens, C.M. (eds.). 2004. *From Source Water to Drinking Water: Workshop Summary.* Institute of Medicine of the National Academies, Washington DC. www.nap.edu.

Revenga, C.; Murray, S.; Abramovitz, J.; Hammond, A. 1998. *Watersheds of the World: Ecological Value and Vulnerability.* Washington DC, World Resources Institute and Worldwatch Institute.

Schopf, JW. 1999. *Cradle of Life: The Discovery of Earth's Earliest Fossils.* Princeton, NJ. Princeton University Press.

Servat, E., et al. 1998. *Water Resources Variability in Africa During the 20th Century.* Wallingford, International Association of Hydrological Sciences. Pub. No. 252.

Shiklomanov, I. 2004. *World Water Resources at the Beginning of the 21st Century.* Cambridge, Cambridge University Press.

———. 2002. *Widespread decline in hydrological monitoring threatens pan-Artic research.* EOS Transactions of the American Geophysical Union. Vol. 83, pp. 13-16.

————. 1998. *Global Renewable Water Resources.* In: H. Zebedi (ed.). *Water: A Looming Crisis?* Proceedings of the International Conference on World Water Resources at the Beginning of the 21st Century. Paris, United Nations Educational, Scientific and Cultural Organization/International Hydrological Programme.

————. 1997. *Comprehensive Assessment of the Freshwater Resources of the World.* Stockholm, Stockholm Environment Institute.

Soussan, J. and Harrison, R. 2000. Commitments on Water Security in the 21st Century: An Analysis of Pledges and Statements at the Ministerial Conference and World Water Forum, The Hague, March 2000.

Swanson P. 2001. *Water: The Drop of Life.* Minnetonka, Minnesota, Northword Press.

Uitto, J.I. and Biswas, A.K. 2000. *Water for Urban Areas: Challenges and Perspectives.* New York, NY, United Nations University Press.

UN (United Nations). 2005a. *Second Committee Recommends Proclamation of International Decade on "Water for Life," 2005-2015.* World Water Day, 22, March 2005. http://www.un.org/NEWSNews/Press/docs/2003/gaef3068.doc.htm.

————. 2005b. *Water for Life Decade: 2005-2015.* United Nations Publication. www.un.org/waterforlifedecade.

————. 2003. *Water for People, Water for Life.* The United Nations World Water Development Report. Paris, UNESCO Publishing.

————. 2002a. *World Population Prospects: The 2000 Revision.* New York, Population Division, Department of Economic and Social Affairs.

————. 2002b. *World Urbanization Prospects: The 2001 Revision; Data Tables and Highlights.* Population Division, New York, Department of Economic and Social Affairs, UN Secretariat, ESA/P/WP/173.

————. 2001. Habitat. *The State of the World's Cities Report 2001.* Nairobi.

————. 2000. *World Urbanization Prospects: The 1999 Revision.* New York.

————. 1992. Agenda 21. Programme of Action for Sustainable Development. Official Outcome of the United Nations Conference on Environment and Development (UNCED), 3–14 June 1992, Rio de Janeiro.

————. 1976. Conference on Human Settlements (Habitat). Recommendation C12 from The Recommendations for National Action endorsed at the UN Conference on Human Settlements in 1976.

UNDP (United Nations Development Programme). 2004. *Protecting International Waters, Sustaining Livelihoods.* www.undp.org/gef.

————. 1997. *Corruption and Good Governance.* MDGD Discussion Paper 3. New York.

UNECE (United Nations Economic Commission for Europe). 2000. *Guidelines on Monitoring and Assessment of Transboundary Groundwaters.* Lelystad.

UNEP (United Nations Environment Programme). 2002. *Water Management.* Industry As a Partner for Sustainable Development Series.

————. 2000. *Global Environmental Outlook 2000.* London, Earthscan Publications.

UNESCO (United Nations Educational, Scientific and Cultural Organization). 2001. *Internationally Shared (Transboundary) Aquifer Resources Management: A Framework Document.* Paris, IHP Non Serial Publications in Hydrology.

———. 1993. *Discharge of Selected Rivers of the World: Mean Monthly and Extreme Discharges.* (1980-1984). Vol. III. Paris, UN Educational, Scientific and Cultural Organization/International Hydrological Programme.

UNFPA (United Nations Population Fund). 2002. *The State of the World Population 2001.* New York.

UNIDO (United Nations Industrial Development Organization). 2002. *Developing Countries Industrial Source Book.* First Edition, Vienna. (Quoted in UN, 2003.)

———. 2001. *Integrated Assessment Management and Governance in River Basins, Coastal Zones and Large Marine Ecosystems.* A UNIDO Strategy Paper. Vienna.

Vorosmarty, C.J., et al. "Global Water Resources: Vulnerability From Climate Change and Population Growth." *Science.* 289.

Walling, D.E. and Webb, B.W. 1996. *Erosion and Sediment Yield. A Global View.* In: D.E. Walling and B.W. Webb (eds.). *Erosion and Sediment Yield: Global and Regional Perspectives.* Wallingford, International Association of Hydrological Sciences. Pub. 236.

Watertech Online. 2001. http://www.watertechonline.com/index.asp.

Water Power and Dam Construction. 1995. *International Water Power and Dam Construction Handbook.* Surrey, Sutton Publishing.

WEC (World Energy Council). 2001. *19th Edition Survey of Energy Resources* (CD-ROM). London.

WHO (World Health Organization). *WHO World Health Report 2002.* Geneva.

———. 2001. *World Development Indicators* (WDI). Washington DC. Available in CD-ROM.

———. 2000. *Water Supply and Sanitation Sector Assessment.* Regional Office for Africa. Harare.

———. 1999a. 'Creating Healthy Cities in the 21st Century'. In: D. Satterthwaite (ed.). *The Earthscan Reader on Sustainable Cities.* London, Earthscan Publications Ltd.

———. 1998. *International Watercourses — Enhancing Cooperation and Managing Conflict.* Technical paper No. 414. Washington DC.

———. 1997. *Guidelines for Drinking-Water Quality.* Second edition. Vol. 3: Surveillance and Control of Community Supplies. Geneva.

———. 1991. *GEMS/Water 1990–2000. The Challenge Ahead.* UNEP/WHO/ UNESCO/WMO Programme on Global Water Quality Monitoring and Assessment. Geneva.

———. 1948. *Statement on Health.* http://www.who.int/en/.

WHO/UNICEF (World Health Organization/United Nations Children's Fund). 2005. *Water For Life: Making It Happen.* Geneva, WHO Press.

————. 2002. *Joint Monitoring Program*. Updated September, 2002.

————. 2000. *Global Water Supply and Sanitation Assessment 2000 Report*. New York.

WMO (World Meteorological Organization). 1999. *Final Report of the Scientific and Technical Committee of the International Decade for Natural Disaster Reduction*. Geneva.

World Bank. 2002. World Development Report 2002: Building Institutions for Markets. Washington DC.

————. 1991. *India Irrigation Sector Review*. Volumes 1 & 2. Washington DC. (Quoted in UN, 2003.)

World Ocean Forum. 2004. *The Ocean, Water, and Public Health: A Common Agenda*. November 15-16, 2004. New York, NY. www.worldoceanforum.org.

WSSCC (World Supply and Sanitation Collaborative Council). 2000. 'Vision 21: A Shared Vision for Hygiene, Sanitation and Water Supply and a Framework for Action'. In: *Proceedings of the Second World Water Forum (The Hague, 17–22 March 2000)*. Geneva.

Zekster, I. and Margat, J. 2004. *Groundwater Resources of the World and Their Use*. Paris, UN Educational, Scientific and Cultural Organization/International Hydrological Programme. Monograph.

European Commission Database on Good Practice in Urban Management and Sustainability

This database, part of the European Commission's site, is designed to help authorities work towards sustainable urban management through the dissemination of good practice and policy.

http://europa.eu.int/comm/urban/

Food and Agriculture Organization (FAO): AQUASTAT

This site provides data on the state of water resources across the world, including an online database on water and agriculture, GIS, maps, etc.

http://www.fao.org/ag/agl/aglw/aquastat/main/

Food and Agriculture Organization (FAO): FAOSTAT

This site includes time series records covering production, trade, food balance sheets, fertilizer and pesticides, land use and irrigation, forest and fishery products, population, agricultural machinery, etc.

http://apps.fao.org/

Food and Agriculture Organization (FAO): Fisheries Global Information System (FIGIS)

This webpage provides global fishery statistics on production, capture production, aquaculture production, fishery commodity production and trade and fishing fleets.

http://www.fao.org/fi/figis/tseries/index.jsp

Food and Agriculture Organization (FAO): Food Insecurity

This site provides information on the state of food insecurity in the world and on global and national efforts.

http://www.fao.org/SOF/sofi/

Food and Agriculture Organization (FAO): World Agriculture Information Center (WAICENT)

FAO's information portal: this is a programme for improving access to documents, statistics, map and multimedia resources.

http://www.fao.org/Waicent/

From Potential Conflict to Co-operation Potential (PCCP)

In collaboration with Green Cross International, and part of the United Nations Educational, Scientific and Cultural Organization's (UNESCO's)

International Hydrological Programme (IHP), PCCP provides tools for aiding conflict resolution in trans-boundary water bodies. PCCP is also a UNESCO contribution to the World Water Assessment Program (WWAP).

http://www.unesco.org/water/wwap/pccp/

Global Water Partnership (GWP)

GWP is a working partnership among all those involved in water management.

http://www.gwpforum.org/

Green Cross International (GCI): Water Conflict Prevention

GCI aims to actively avoid and mitigate conflict in water-stressed regions. This site provides news events, links and a bibliography.

http://gcinwa.newaccess.ch/index.htm

Health Politics

This site addresses complex health policy issues that impact health consumers and their caregivers.

http://www.healthpolitics.com

International Water Law Project

A Joint United Nations initiative, the international water law project provides information, a bibliography and documents on water laws relating to trans-boundary water resources.

http://www.internationalwaterlaw.org/

International Water Management Institute (IWMI)

The IWMI deals with issues related to water management and food security: water for agriculture; ground water; poverty; rural developments; policy and institutions; health and environment.

http://www.cgiar.org/iwmi/

International Water Management Institute (IWMI): Water for Agriculture

This site provides information on issues related to water for agriculture: research activities, list of publications and links. This site is part of a larger site that houses information on a plethora of water management-related topics, such as the environment, health, etc.

http://www.cgiar.org/iwmi/agriculture/

United Nations Convention to Combat Desertification (UNCCD)

This webpage includes topics related to desertification, while staying in the context of sustainable development.

http://www.unccd.int/

United Nations Framework Convention on Climate Change (UNFCCC)

Part of the United Nations (UN) framework, this site provides information relating to flood management and flood disaster reduction.

http://www.unfccc.int/

Society for the Promotion of Area Resource Centres (SPARC)

SPARC is a non-governmental organization devoted to working with the urban poor.

The site provides information on projects, news events, publications and related links, including information on the National Slum Dwellers Federation (NSDF).
http://www.sparcindia.org/

Transboundary Freshwater Dispute Database

This site includes a searchable database of water-related treaties organized by basin, countries or states involved. It focuses on problems related to international waters.

http://www.transboundarywaters.orst.edu/

UN-Habitat: Global Urban Observatory

Part of the UN Habitat site, this section provides policy-oriented urban indicators, statistics and other information on global urban conditions and trends.

http://www.unchs.org/programmes/guo

United Children's Fund (UNICEF) Statistics: Water and Sanitation

This site contains UNICEF's key statistical database with detailed country-specific information that was used for the end-of-decade assessment. Among the main themes are Water and Sanitation, Child Survival and Health, Child Nutrition, Maternal Health, Education, Child Rights.

http://www.childinfo.org/eddb/water.htm

United Nations Convention on Biological Diversity (UNCBD)

The UNCBD promotes nature and human well-being, focusing on the importance of biological diversity for the health of people and the planet.

http://www.biodiv.org

United Nations Development Programme (UNDP)

The UNDP is the UN's global development network, advocating for change and connecting countries to knowledge, experience and resources to help people build a better life.

http://www.undp.org/

United Nations Development Programme (UNDP): Public-Private Partnerships for the Urban Environment (PPPUE)

The PPPUE supports the development of public-private partnerships at the local level in order to ensure more sustainable urban management practices. The aim is to facilitate meeting the challenges faced by cities in providing basic services to populations.

http://www.undp.org/ppp/

United Nations Environment Programme (UNEP): Floods and Droughts

This site includes strategies, links, documents and other resources for coping with flood and drought.

http://freshwater.unep.net/index.cfm?issue=water_flood_drought

United Nations Environment Programme (UNEP): Freshwater

Information on the key issues of the global water situation are available on

this webpage. One section is dedicated to water and ecosystems.
http://freshwater.unep.net/

United Nations Environment Programme (UNEP): Global Environment Monitoring System (GEMS/WATER)
GEMS/WATER is a multifaceted water science programme oriented towards understanding fresh water quality issues throughout the world.
http://www.gemswater.org/

United Nations International Strategy for Disaster Reduction (ISDR)
This international site provides information, news events and training courses in order to increase awareness of the importance of disaster reduction.
http://www.unisdr.org/

World Bank: Urban Development
This site is committed to promoting sustainable cities by improving the lives of the poor. This department of the World Bank provides inter alia information on a variety of aspects of urban management.
http://www.worldbank.org/urban/

World Bank: Law Resource Center
This resource center offers an organized database of links and tools on international organizations, laws, treaties and laws of nations with links to their constitutions and legislation.
http://www4.worldbank.org/legal/lawlibrary.html

World Health Organization (WHO): Healthy Cities and Urban Governance
This site provides information on health issues in urban areas, as well as ideas on making cities healthier, news events from around the world and links to related sites.
http://www.who.dk/eprise/main/WHO/Progs/HCP/Home

World Health Organization (WHO): Statistical Information System (WHOSIS)
This site includes a guide to health and health-related epidemiological and statistical information available from WHO and elsewhere.
http://www3.who.int/whosis/menu.cfm

World Health Organization (WHO): Water, Sanitation and Health Programme
Regularly updated information of the WHO's Programme on Water, Sanitation and Health, including all publications and documents in PDF and HTML format files.
http://www.who.int/water_sanitation_health

World Health Organization/Pan-American Health Organization/Pan-American Centre for Sanitary Engineering and Environmental Sciences (WHO/PAHO/CEPIS) Virtual Library on Health and the Environment: Assessment of Drinking Water and Sanitation in the Americas
This site provides data and indicators on urban and rural population, water, sanitation, general health and hygiene.
http://www.cepis.ops-oms.org/enwww/eva2000/infopais.html

World Health Organization/United Children's Fund (WHO/UNICEF) Joint Monitoring Programme for Water Supply and Sanitation (JMP)
Data is available on this webpage on access to water supply and sanitation services at the country, regional and global levels.
http://www.wssinfo.org

World Meteorological Organization (WMO): Global Runoff Data Centre (GRDC)
The GRDC offers a collection and dissemination of river discharge data on a global scale.
http://grdc.bafg.de/servlet/is/Entry.987.Display/

World Meteorological Organization (WMO): Hydrology and Water Resources Programme
This site includes a collection and analysis of hydrological data as a basis for assessing and managing fresh water resources.
http://www.wmo.ch/web/homs/

World Meteorological Organization (WMO): World Climate Research Programme (WCRP)
This site includes studies of the global atmosphere, oceans, sea and land ice and the land surface, which together constitute the Earth's physical climate system.
http://www.wmo.ch/web/wcrp/wcrp-home.html

World Meteorological Organization (WMO): World Hydrological Observing System (WHYCOS)
WHYCOS is a global network of national hydrological observatories.
http://www.wmo.ch/web/homs/projects/whycos.html

World Meteorological Organization (WMO)/Global Water Partnership (GWP): The Associated Programme on Flood Management (APFM)
This site promotes flood management within the context of Integrated Water Resources Management.
http://www.wmo.ch/apfm/

World Resources Institute (WRI): EarthTrends
This site is an environmental Information Portal. Among the issues featured are coastal and marine ecosystems, water resources and fresh water ecosystems, human health and well-being, biodiversity and protected areas.
http://earthtrends.wri.org/

World Water Assessment Programme / United Nations Educational, Scientific and Cultural Organization (WWAP/UNESCO): Water Portal
This portal is a new initiative for accessing and sharing water data and information from all over the world.
http://www.unesco.org/water/wwap/index.shtml

Worldwide Fund for Nature (WWF): The Living Planet
The Living Planet Report is WWF's periodic update on the state of the world's ecosystems and the human pressures on them through the consumption of renewable natural resources.
http://www.panda.org/livingplanet/

The Ocean, Water
& Public Health:
A Common Agenda

Based on the findings of the inaugural World Ocean Forum
November 15–16, 2004, New York, New York, www.worldoceanforum.org

The ocean plays a crucial role in a variety of natural processes, including, among many others, fresh water distribution and climatological events which have a direct and lasting impact on the health of human communities around the world. Looking at this theme *from the land* requires that we understand that the ocean is not "a place apart," but rather an essential part of the process of life: the hydrologic cycle, the food cycle and the biodiversity requisite to understanding natural systems and their adaptation to human need. Looking at this theme *from the sea* requires that we understand that solutions to critical ocean problems must be implemented on the land where the impact of population growth, agricultural and industrial development and human misunderstanding and indifference are challenging the ocean's capacity for self-healing.

Our Assumptions
- The ocean is an inclusive global, social and political ecosystem — the ocean affects each of us and we affect the ocean every day. In order to truly improve understanding, we must broaden the education base — including educating patients and families, amending medical school curricula, engaging nurses and pharmacists and building strategic alliances at all levels.
- Everything needs to be thought of — and communicated — in terms of public health.

Trends and Developments
- The world's oceans are overstressed and clean water is growing more scarce. But, there is room for hope if we act now.
- Recent discoveries of unique ocean life provide tangible values through biomedical advances. And, as other advances in technology are increasingly available, the supply of investment money that could be devoted to water in the private equity sector has grown exponentially.

Our Vision
- Access to safe, clean water and basic sanitation for all human beings
- Recovery of the ocean environment through mitigation and change to provide the maximum benefit to human health.

Our Challenge
- There has already been much work done by many brilliant minds. The challenge ahead is not to re-evaluate what was or must be done, but to find areas where there is broad consensus among diverse constituencies and move forward together.
- In the frantic pace of today's world, there is a shortage of time to think and to act. And, while much research remains to deepen our understanding of the world's oceans, there is much that we already know and can act on immediately.

Our Opportunity
- The international *Water for Life* decade begins in 2005, officially designated by the United Nations as an attempt to cut in half the number of people who are unable to reach or afford safe drinking water and who do not have access to basic sanitation.
- A distinguished group of leaders from more than 15 countries, including medical doctors and research scientists, non-governmental organization (NGO) representatives, public health officials, business leaders and government officials crafted a succinct list of ideas to be pursued by both human scientists and physical scientists in the years ahead.
- It is their hope that the following ideas will achieve these strategic expectations, ultimately reaching an audience of millions around the world, and contributing to the immediate solution of critical problems and to positive change.

LEADERSHIP RECOMMENDATIONS

"Health is not owned by the governments...civil society will have to play a big role in this."
—Dr. Kerstin Leitner, World Health Organization

Coordinate and consolidate diverse partnerships to leverage existing resources

First Win
- Develop partnerships and alliances with the World Medical Association, World Ocean Observatory and Pfizer Medical Humanities Initiative, as well as National Oceanic and Atmospheric Administration (NOAA), the United Nations and the World Health Organization

Additional Actions
- Create a "network of networks" and a basis for public discourse and education about oceans, water and public health
- Engage private sector for advancement of ocean, water and public health issues
- Develop a global business coalition for the oceans, water and public health
- Institute a framework to foster cooperation among governments, nongovernmental organizations, physicians and scientists with respect to conservation and sustainable use of ocean resources
- Encourage civic associations to engage their local chapters in efforts to improve the supply of fresh, clean water to communities who lack it

Capitalize on innovation and new technologies to expand access to clean water

First Win
- Encourage patient and consumer use of high-impact, low-cost, point-of-use filtration for drinking water

Additional Action
- Identify additional cost-effective technologies such as low-flow toilets and UV wastewater treatment systems

Conduct research to support decision-making systems and communications efforts

First Win
- Support strategic actions to counter the negative impacts of toxins in coastal waters, including research analysis of organohalogens, heavy metals and inorganic compounds

Additional Actions
- Advocate augmented research activities and communications efforts concerning the ocean's biomedical potential to government agencies, international organizations and the private sector
- Define and establish a physician/pharmacist/nurse sentinel surveillance system — a mechanism for health professionals to continually gather data based on indicators that, when triggered, should illuminate concerns within the health system
- Support aquaculture and genetic engineering as ways to produce bulk supplies of chemicals for biomedical research

Guide and support community-building efforts to increase capacity and improve efficiency

First Win

- Explore ways to control and regulate the drilling of wells and installation of septic tank systems in the context of public health

Additional Actions

- Strive for sustainable development using existing municipal controls — such as licensing or zoning — as a cost-effective alternative to industrial treatment
- Replicate smaller models throughout the world to duplicate successes while avoiding problems associated with upscaling
- Increase scientific training through investing in infrastructure, education and equipment in order to increase global research capabilities and enact long-term and sustainable development in host countries
- Build alliances with other organizations to advocate for smart growth to sprawl reduction
- Further support current drug-discovery programs, such as those by the International Cooperative Biodiversity Group, in biodiversity-rich areas that are economically poor

Advocate for effective ocean and water policy

First Win

- Use Harmful Algal Blooms (HABs) to inform local policymakers of need to deal with basic sanitation and safety issues

Additional Actions

- Conduct a survey of local elected officials and policymakers to identify potential champions for ocean resource development
- Support the development of "quiet zones" that would range from simple no-fishing zones to fully fledged marine protected areas

"If we could put the best available science into practice — and communicate effectively — we could get a lot done."
—Dr. Jonathan Quick, Management Sciences for Health

Implement targeted education efforts to inform key stakeholder groups

First Win

- Distribute educational pocket-sized guides about ocean-friendly seafood and other nutritional information for patients and consumers through public health officials and secondary schools

Additional Actions

- Seek funding to launch comprehensive education programs for developing nations to help decrease contamination of water and increase access to quality water
- Alter medical school curricula to include more oceans and water courses
- Create paid internships and summer jobs for first- and second-year medical students
- Change the framing and perception of environmental actions as public health actions
- Organize an informal speakers' bureau for health organization meetings and conferences to inform and educate about water and ocean issues

Create evidence-based, politically astute communications packages to improve awareness and generate interest in oceans and water issues especially among health professionals

First Wins

- Approach medical publications — such as *JAMA* — for a theme issue on water and oceans
- Create a communications plan to be used for the international Water for Life decade (2005–2015)

Additional Actions

- Create templates that communicate the value of water to patients and consumers in useful formats such as bill inserts, mass transit advertising campaigns and pocket-sized brochures
- Formalize an *Oceans for Health* network of professional communicators
- Create "mind-maps" on why physicians and patients should be interested in these issues

The World Ocean Forum — a rare opportunity for leading scientists and policy experts from the public and private sectors to engage in such close discussion of vital issues — was made possible by a partnership between the World Medical Association, World Ocean Observatory and the Pfizer Medical Humanities Initiative.

World Ocean Forum Participants

(Note: This list indicates the organizational affiliations of participants at the time of the World Ocean Forum.)

Enrique Accorsi, MD
Health Commission of the Chilean Parliament

Tundi Agardy, PhD
Sound Seas

Franklin Apfel, MD
World Health Communication Associates

James Appleyard, MD
World Medical Association

Hans Kristian Bakke, MD
Norwegian Medical Association

Jaroslav Blahos, MD
Czech Medical Association

Marcia M. Brewster
United Nations

Robin Buchannon, PhD
National Institute for Undersea Science and Technology

Philip Burgess
National Oceans Office, Australia

Sarah Chasis, JD
Natural Resources Defense Council

Yank Coble, MD
World Medical Association

Christine Coussens, PhD
Institute of Medicine

Peter Davidson
Davidson Media Group

F. Ronald Denham, PhD
Rotary International

Paula Diperna
World Ocean Observatory

John T. Everett, PhD
National Oceanic and Atmospheric Administration

William Gerwick, PhD
Oregon State University

Vladimir Golitsyn, PhD
United Nations

Peter Harrison, PhD
National Research Council of Canada

Glen Hiemstra
Futurist.com

A. Judson Hill
Halifax Group

Ton Hoek
International Pharmaceutical Federation

Delon Human, MD
World Medical Association

Lawrence S. Huntington
Fiduciary Trust Company International

Otmar Kloiber, MD
World Medical Association

Kerstin Leitner, PhD
World Health Organization

Kgosi Letlape, MD
South African Medical Association

Mike Magee, MD
Pfizer Medical Humanities Initiative

Peter McCarthy, PhD
Harbor Branch Oceanographic Institution

Richard Medley, PhD
Medley Global Advisors

Bill Mott
The Ocean Project

Peter Neill
World Ocean Observatory

Judith Oulton, RN
International Council of Nurses

Roger Payne, PhD
The Ocean Alliance and The Whale Conservation Institute

Michael Burke Phillips, QC
Canada's Department of Foreign Affairs

Jonathan Quick, MD
Management Sciences for Health

Anne H. Rogers
United Nations

Albert Schumacher, MD
Canadian Medical Association

Randy Smoak, MD
American Medical Association

Lisa Speer
Natural Resources Defense Council

Richard W. Spinrad, PhD
National Oceanic and Atmospheric Administration

Juha Uitto, PhD
United Nations Development Programme

Christopher Ward
New York City Department of Environmental Protection

John Wellner
Ontario Medical Association

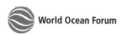

World Ocean Forum

The World Medical Association (WMA) is an international organization representing physicians. It was founded on 17 September 1947, when physicians from 27 different countries met at the First General Assembly of the WMA in Paris. The organization was created to ensure the independence of physicians, and to work for the highest possible standards of ethical behavior and care by physicians, at all times. The WMA provides a forum for its member associations to communicate freely, to co-operate actively, to achieve consensus on high standards of medical ethics and professional competence, and to promote the professional freedom of physicians worldwide. This unique partnership facilitates high-calibre, humane care to patients in a healthy environment, enhancing the quality of life for all people in the world.

WORLD OCEAN **Observatory**

The World Ocean Observatory is a central place of exchange for ocean information, education and public discourse. South Street Seaport Museum is developing an Internet-based program to expand public awareness of the implication of the ocean for the future of human life. The ocean demands a new information service that meets the needs of an inquisitive public and transcends the limits of governments, research organizations, national interests and non-governmental organizations with more narrowly defined environmental agendas.

Pfizer Medical
Humanities Initiative

The Pfizer Medical Humanities Initiative is a research and educational program committed to the study and enhancement of the patient-physician relationship in the United States and around the world. Since it was funded in 1997, the initiative has provided significant support through scholarships, grants and awards that strengthen the medical profession and enhance the relationship patients have with their physicians and other caregivers. For more information, visit www.positiveprofiles.com.

"Access to safe water is a fundamental human need

and therefore a basic human right."

—*Kofi Annan, United Nations Secretary General*

APPENDIX II 25 Water Facts Everyone Should Know

1. Water is essential to all life.
2. Oceans, surface water and ground water are interconnected and interdependent.
3. Most of the Earth's water (99%+) is not fresh, not accessible, or neither fresh nor accessible.
4. Humans need 2.3 liters of water on average per day to survive. Humans' average daily diet however derives from an investment of 3,000 liters of water.
5. Agriculture is the leading consumer of water worldwide, consuming 70% of our fresh water.
6. Irrigated fields have 400% greater food yield than rain fed fields. By 2030, 70% of the world's grain crop will come from irrigated fields
7. Currently 27% of fish consumed by humans is "grown" through aquaculture. China alone is responsible for 70% of the "crop."
8. Industry is the second leading consumer of fresh water, consuming 22% of our total supply worldwide.
9. Water is essential for all forms of energy generation worldwide.
10. Global hydropower currently provides about 20% of our energy worldwide.
11. Supplies of safe, fresh water are declining and global population is increasing. In the past 100 years our population has tripled, and water consumption has increased six-fold.
12. Water scarcity is increasingly common. 3.4 billion global citizens will live in water-scarce areas by 2025.
13. One-sixth (17%) of humans lack fresh, safe water and two-fifths (40%) lack adequate sanitation.
14. Investment in water and sanitation has a 34-fold return on investment.
15. Watershed catchbasins cover 45% of Earth's land and support 60% of our global population.
16. 145 nations share a catchbasin with another nation.
17. Urban environments, usually associated with catchbasin areas, continue to grow and will house 60% of our population by 2025.
18. Safety and security of urban populations are fundamentally dependent on wise water management.

19. Surface water in the developing world is the dumping ground for 70% of industrial waste and 90% of local raw sewage.

20. Water-related diseases account for 25% of all deaths worldwide and 50% of all hospitalized patients.

21. Water-related disasters between 1990 and 2000 claimed over half a million lives. Most could have been prevented by Integrated Water Resource Management and Disaster Preparedness.

22. Global warming is a significant contributor to water scarcity and water disasters.

23. Integrated Water Resource Management (IWRM) is organized at the catchment level, proactively balancing infrastructure development, allocations of water and mitigation of risk.

24. IWRM has social, political and economic dimensions that directly impact human health, poverty levels and gender equality.

25. IWRM requires reliable data and careful valuation of water as a resource. Identifying true cost of provisions of safe water and sanitation is essential for financing and creating sustainable and reliable infrastructure.